Birthing

The Easy Way

By someone who learned the hard way

Sheila Stubbs

Reprinted 2008

Birthing the Easy Way
P.O. Box 161
Springford, ON   N0J 1X0
Canada

Printed and bound in Canada, eh?

Birthing the Easy Way

By someone who learned the hard way

Sheila Stubbs

ACKNOWLEDGEMENTS

I am indebted to La Leche League, for the dedicated mothers who devote their time to help others learn the womanly art of breastfeeding. They showed me the difference between happily nursing a child and merely lactating.

To Terry, who traveled with me from a La Leche League meeting on the road to emotional healing from surgical birth, and was present to welcome both my daughters into the world amidst squeals of joy;

To Joanne, who gave me the privilege of being present when she welcomed *her* daughter into the world, and let me see first-hand how to birth the easy way;

To the memory of Marilyn Moran, who encouraged me to go "all the way,"

And to Bert, who took me there.

Birthing the Easy Way

... by someone who learned the hard way

Sheila Stubbs

First Base

CHAPTER 1

Getting Lucky

A single white shoelace for tying the cord was the only thing we had ready for the baby's birth. We delivered him by the soft light of our bedroom lamp in the wee hours of a cold February morning while a blizzard raged outside.

"You're so lucky," my neighbour said later the same day when she came to investigate the news of a baby being born in the neighborhood. "You're one of the lucky women who have an easy time when you give birth."

Lucky? I thought. *Just plain lucky*? My first baby was born by cesarean after 21 hours of labour because the doctors said my pelvis was too small to deliver an eight-pound baby safely. Was I lucky then? According to some people, I was: Lucky to have doctors who could do this life-saving surgery, lucky to have a healthy baby, and lucky to have avoided the pain of childbirth. Avoided pain? Pain was not avoided: pain from the surgery lasted six weeks.

"One of the lucky women who have an easy time," my neighbour had said. The obstetrician who performed the cesarean section told me I had an inadequate pelvis. He said I might consider attempting a natural birth only if he was certain I was having a smaller baby. Under his strict guidelines and in carefully controlled conditions, he guessed I had about a 30% chance of having a vaginal birth… if I was lucky.

Contrary to the doctor's prediction, I beat his odds when two years later I had a VBAC — Vaginal Birth After Cesarean — with a *bigger* baby. It was a "natural" birth but it was *not* "an easy time" as my neighbour had said. *Give birth easily*? Dealing with 28 hours of back labour, and over two hours of pushing, straining so hard my face turned purple, small blood vessels burst around my eyes and my ears were popping was *not* easy. I was in agony, exhausted, suffered a perineal tear, and even begged the doctor to use forceps to save me from further torture. Hell itself, I thought, could not be much worse! *Lucky*?

No, luck did not bring me to gentle birth any more than my neighbour was lucky to have a nice home and a good job. It took some planning to accomplish and reap the benefits, both for her and for me. Maybe some people are born lucky, but not me. I had to learn how to give birth easily and I learned the hard way.

According to my obstetrician, my cesarean section was required due to fetal distress as a result of cephalo-pelvic disproportion. In layman's terms it means the 8-½ pound baby was in trouble because he couldn't fit through my small pelvic bones. But when my next baby, weighing over 10 pounds, was born vaginally and without any drugs, forceps or other manipulation, I realized there was nothing wrong with my pelvis after all! There must have been something else wrong; something else causing a perfectly healthy mother to require surgery to deliver a perfectly healthy baby.

I began to mistrust the whole system which declares childbirth to be a risky, dangerous medical problem. I never went back to the hospital for delivery again, and the rest of my babies — four more — have been born at home.

But isn't it terribly risky? Isn't home birth dangerous? Am I just plain *lucky* nothing has gone wrong?

I am only 5' 3½" tall and of an average build. (Well, OK, I'm on the plump side!) Only one of my babies was smaller than the cesarean-born baby, but he was a month premature. We didn't go to the hospital for his birth either.

According to most obstetricians, my circumstances would put me into a High-Risk category, necessitating close monitoring in a hospital. These include all of the following:

- previous miscarriage
- previous cesarean section
- premature birth
- previous child weighing over nine pounds
- bleeding during pregnancy
- fifth or later child
- "android pelvis"
- Rh incompatibility
- premature rupture of membranes

I repeat, I have experienced all of the above, and still had easy, problem-free home births.

Lucky. Was I really just *lucky*?

The cesarean section, without a doubt, is a life-saving operation. But, the rate of cesarean sections is 30% or more. Why? How can doctors justify one in four women needing surgery to get the baby safely out? They can't, unless they could prove a 30% morbidity/mortality rate in places without access to cesarean. And of the remaining 70% who have a vaginal birth: how many women can actually give birth with no interventions — no IV, no drugs, no forceps, no stitches?

You might be wondering: Would we even want to give birth without these interventions? Wouldn't childbirth be more dangerous? Wouldn't babies suffer more damage? Doesn't medical intervention help women avoid needless suffering and prevent babies from damage? Can the average woman cope without some pain medication?"

Or is medical intervention actually part of the problem?

I have a typical newspaper clipping in my collection; a front-page article about a young woman who gave birth by accident at home. She called 911 when she knew she wasn't going to make it to the hospital, and a police officer arrived to find her already giving birth. He caught the baby and then an ambulance took her and the baby to the hospital where they met with news reporters. The baby had been *breech*. In the hospital most, if not all, breech babies are delivered by cesarean. But here was a frightened, totally unprepared woman at home, with a non-medical person attending her, and she had a quick, normal, vaginal birth. The doctor's comment was, of course, "She was extremely fortunate."[1]

I had a premature baby at home. I had babies over ten pounds at home. I had meconium staining. I had a previous cesarean. I had premature rupture of the membranes. Obstetricians consider all these factors to be to be risks requiring obstetrical management. All were handled with no problems at home. Was it because I was lucky?

The Guinness Book of World Records documents the world's most prolific mother was a Mrs. Vassilyev, who gave birth to 69 children. She also holds the world record for the largest number of multiple births. In a 40-year span, Mrs. Vassilyev had 27 pregnancies in which she gave birth to — you ready for this? — 16 pairs of twins, *seven* sets of *triplets*, and *four sets of quadruplets!!*

The amazing part of this story to me is this: only two of those 69 children failed to survive past their infancy. These births occurred in the 1700's, long before we had obstetricians, pediatricians, incubators, and neonatal intensive care units, all of which we "know" are essential to ensure survival in such as high-risk situation as a multiple birth.

Maybe she was just "lucky." Sixty-nine times over.

(I don't know if I would consider myself "lucky" to be blessed with two-year old twins while diapering one-year-old triplets, while pregnant with quadruplets. This was a Russian peasant woman, not the wife of some wealthy emperor who could hire help.)

The famous Dionne quintuplets were born in a rural farmhouse in Ontario with no electricity or running water. All five babies survived as we know, and the mother went on to have more children.

A woman in Titusville, Florida wrote a book about her experience giving birth alone by choice. Disgusted with her childbirth experience in the hospital with her first two children, when she "screamed and writhed and chewed [her] fingers bloody,[2]" Mrs. Carter thereafter chose to retreat to her own bedroom to give birth all alone. She had seven babies by herself. Was she just lucky?

Lucky might be the woman who doesn't even know she's in labour until the baby nearly falls out! She feels no pain, doesn't even realize her baby is coming until it's in her underpants. I'm not *that* lucky!

Some women seem to be blessed with a Body Built Best for Birthing Babies and can pop 'em out like watermelon seeds. My friend Joanne is an example. They broke her water to induce labour and in *twenty-one minutes* the baby was in her arms! It's probably hereditary: Joanne herself was born in the lobby of the hospital which was as far as her mother got when Joanne made her appearance — and they lived across the road from the hospital!

I did not have painless births, but I did learn how to have easier births. They are easy in the sense that I am up and walking around during labour right up until the pushing stage, then bustling about like normal immediately after the birth too. I don't have any exceptional pain tolerance or stamina and I'm certainly no athlete. My only aerobic exercise would be what one gets climbing a mountain of laundry every day or running to catch a two year old who's just found a black marker pen. During pregnancy my weight gain has been as little as 17 pounds as much as 50+ pounds. I'm just plain old average normal.

I learned giving birth is much less painful when you are not afraid of it. You don't need to take classes to be taught how to breathe or do special exercises. You don't need to have enormous hips. And you don't need a lot of medical technology. All you need is some basic information, common sense, confidence, and faith in your own body's ability to give birth.

Even if you have no confidence now, don't give up! What little confidence I started out with was surgically removed somehow with my c-section. How could I believe in my ability to give birth when my body had failed to do its job? How could I possibly have any faith in myself when I needed doctors to rescue my baby from my body? Even dumb weasels and squirrels and caribou can get their babies out without an operation, but I couldn't.

The decision to give birth at home in spite of the risks was not made on a whim. It would be crazy to make such a critical decision without doing any research.

> "Hey Honey, the doctor said I have an abnormally shaped, small pelvis and will never be able to deliver a normal-sized child. He said there's a good chance the scar on my uterus will burst open, and the baby and I will both bleed to death before your eyes. What the heck — let's have the baby at home just for fun!"

Some people believe women in tribal cultures have an easier time than we do. I don't know whether or not this is true. I do know that statistically, in spite of technological progress in North America, the mortality rate is much better in other countries. Holland, Denmark, Norway, Sweden and Italy, for example, all have peri-natal mortality rates *less than half* of Canada's rate.[3] The rates are even worse in the U.S.

Really, with our Health Care system and affluent living conditions here in North America we have no excuse for such a poor mortality rate. We have every opportunity to be well-nourished, healthy, educated and live in comfortable homes. For being born in a wealthy nation at least, we should consider ourselves *lucky*.

CHAPTER 2

Taking Control

> The biggest problem facing a pregnant woman is not nausea or fatigue or her wardrobe – it's free advice. I learned very quickly to agree with everyone. I would smile and say, "Of course, you are so right. What an excellent idea!" Then I would go on doing whatever I knew to be right for my baby. Everyone was happy.
>
> - Sophia Loren

One of the goals of childbirth education classes is to teach what happens to your body during the process of labour and delivery because a basic understanding of anatomy and physiology helps reduce fear and therefore, pain. A woman with no idea about what is happening will be more afraid and tense than the woman who understands what her body is doing, why it hurts, and that it is a normal process.

What many childbirth education classes overlook, however, is the pleasant side of childbirth.

Pleasant? Childbirth is *pleasant? Pain* is pleasant?

Let's look at an analogy for a moment. Suppose for a moment that all you knew about the beach was what a horrible, dirty place it is to visit: sand gets in your shoes, the dead fish stink, and seagulls fly overheard dropping bombs on you. If you knew nothing else about the beach, you'd stay away. But instead of the negative aspects we focus on how much fun it is to play in the waves and to dig our toes into the sand. We remember the refreshing scent of the sea. We welcome the therapeutic effects of basking in the warm sun while the rhythmic sound of the waves helps us unwind. Likewise, we also need to hear about the positive side of childbirth, not just about the relentless pain, the unknown dangers, potential risks and horror stories of dead or damaged babies. We rarely hear about the good stuff, and I don't mean just the "healthy baby" outcome. I mean the journey itself, not just the destination.

It's like swimming. Swimming, like childbirth, can carry risks, so we have a healthy respect for it. Again, imagine what it would be like if all you ever heard about swimming was how dangerous it was. Imagine if the TV show *Baywatch* had showed only the dangerous rescues, the near-drownings, and the people screaming for help, but never the beautiful sunny beach, the surfers having fun, or the stunning bikini-clad women. You would have a totally different view of the beach life, seeing swimming as a very risky activity.

Imagine what it would be like in this scenario if lifeguards across the continent united to form a powerful organization to help spread the message about the dangers of swimming unsupervised. They set up an intense training course covering all aspects of swimming and in-depth study of water. With this increase in knowledge and the power of their organization behind them, they become the guardians of all waterways, working together to warn people of the terrible risks involved in swimming. The public is discouraged from swimming in backyard pools and urged instead to come to public pools for their own safety. There they can be closely watched by trained lifeguards, where resuscitation equipment is readily available in case of accidents.

Soon, everyone becomes afraid of waterways. The media helps spread the word with reports of drownings in lakes and rivers, reminding us that these deaths would not have occurred in a public swimming facility. Magazines feature stories written by lifeguards, where they offer swimming tips and answer reader's questions, and the science of swimming begins to sound very complicated indeed. You begin to hear stories on TV from people who had a horrible time swimming, and how the lifeguard saved their life. The experts talk about the frigid water, the dangers of hypothermia and cramps. You almost wonder why in the world anyone would ever want to swim. What if something goes wrong?

We teach our children to be afraid of the water, and they wouldn't dare go near it without a lifeguard present. When children ask about swimming, parents avoid telling them anything, lest they frighten them, as they learned on the "Ask a Lifeguard" reality show. "Never mind," they would say reassuringly, "The lifeguard will take care of you when it comes time to swim."

Swimming, something people have always done with happy anticipation, confidence, and a healthy respect for the known risks, now has become something to fear. In fact, you could be put in jail for failing to seek a lifeguard's services for your swim!

Staying Afloat

Despite the fear of swimming, most people choose to swim across the river once or twice during their lives. It's like a rite of passage, when they gain respect and prove their maturity and courage

"Have your swims close together," people say, "and get it over with."

Some people don't want to merely get across the river; they would like their swim to be a "good experience." These folks take swimming education classes to teach them all about the river, the water, and how to prepare for the swim. On dry land they are taught different swim strokes and will practice their strokes and breathing exercises every day. Classes taught at public swimming pools tend to focus on how to co-operate best with the lifeguards and the use of lifesaving equipment, while independent classes might focus more on how to swim by your own strength.

Not everyone has the same river experience because there are so many variables in the river swim. Some people take their swim on a sunny day when the water is unusually calm and warm and the current carries you easily to the other side. Other times the current is so strong you fear being swept away. Some swimmers must fight against the wind and waves with every stroke. A few people, for reasons we don't understand, just can't seem to float, but this is rare, and in these situations we are grateful for the lifeguard heroes.

Many people find out as much as they can about the current where they live. Some travel farther upriver where the water is calmer or the lifeguards have newer, better equipment. It's wise to check out your lifeguard. Is he the type who likes to have all his swimmers hooked up to the lifeboat just in case, or is he the type to coach you to the shore where he helps you into a big warm towel? Some have the newest technology available to monitor your swim, others are more old-fashioned.

One fact we all accept without question is that *the majority of lifeguards have never actually been in the water themselves!* Lifeguards study for years to qualify for the job. They have a wealth of knowledge and experience around water and they are well armed with rescuing equipment, but have no idea what swimming actually feels like. That doesn't matter to them, because their job is not to make the swim enjoyable but to make sure it's safe. The only way they can assure the safety of the swim is if they control the swimmer.

The lifeguard has a high-speed motor boat filled with life rings, various sizes of lifejackets, water wings, and ropes. There are foam boards, snorkels, masks, flippers, an oxygen tank, resuscitation equipment, a gun (to shoot the sharks, just in case), towels, blankets, re-hydration drinks, sunscreen, and other items they keep secret, because you aren't qualified to know, unless you are a lifeguard. The best lifeguards use newest technology to insure nothing goes wrong, including a wireless monitor to record heart rate, breathing rate and body temperature.

Taking Control

Everyone is pretty nervous when you go into the water, hoping and praying nothing goes wrong. The lifeguard throws you in the water to help speed things up a bit. The cold water takes your breath away. Engine roaring, the lifeguard drives circles around you so he can keep a close eye on you. This causes waves to splash over your face, leaving you sputtering and coughing.

Your coach accompanies the lifeguard in the boat along with a team of well-trained assistants who are there to help you in the event something goes wrong. They shout out instructions on the proper way to move your arms and legs and will reprimand you if you are not doing it correctly. The Australian crawl is the only swimstroke permitted. Your coach's job is to remind you to breathe, because you might forget.

Based on studies done on thousands of swimmers, lifeguards have determined you should be able to swim at a certain rate of speed. The lifeguards warn you of the increased risks of swimming too slowly. You could get too fatigued and drown. You could develop hypothermia and drown. You could get muscle cramps and drown.

Halfway across you are tired and flustered and having a hard time keeping up even though your coach is helping you as much as he can, yelling *Stroke! Stroke!* You wanted to swim "naturally" but this is just too hard! The lifeguard finally helps you. As you sputter for air he stuffs you into a lifejacket, which is attached with ropes and hooks to the boat. What relief! The lifejacket helps you relax and enjoy the river, since you no longer have to struggle to stay afloat. It's cumbersome though, and slows you down even more.

The lifeguard is glad you are roped to the boat, so he will now be able to drag you safely behind. If necessary he may decide to haul you right into the boat. Some swimmers are extremely disappointed if this happens, but the lifeguard assures them there are just some cases where the boat ride is the safest option. "What's important is not whether you took the boat or swam," the lifeguard reminds you, "Your goal was to get across the river, and that's all that matters."

Some folks criticize the lifeguards for this statement, saying they just want to hurry you up so they can get to their Wednesday afternoon Beach Volleyball game. It's unfair, because after all, the lifeguard cares about your safety and does his best to help make your swim as secure and comfortable as possible. Don't forget, in the old days before lifeguards, sometimes people drowned!

In spite of the safety features in place, some people still drown. They may have gotten too close to the motorboat, or got caught themselves caught in the ropes, or any number of things that can go wrong. But at least they know the Lifeguards did everything they could.

Occasionally, there are accidents when someone falls in a river unsupervised and actually swims across the river alone! Wow! The news crews rush in to interview them. How could this happen? You swam by yourself? How did you manage? How did you know what to do? Weren't you scared?

The news story invariably ends with a statement from a lifeguard. "They were extremely fortunate," the lifeguard reminds us, with a look of grave concern.

What's worse is that we've even heard there are some crazy fools who *plan* to swim across the river alone! They prepare their own towels, snorkel and flippers and generally keep quiet about it, because they know people whisper about them, talking about how dangerous and stupid it is to risk your life in such a careless manner. These brave swimmers don't make it to the newspaper headlines though. There's nothing sensational to report but a quiet little swim across the river. Besides, the media can't understand it. How can they do it, just like it was the most natural thing in the world?

I confess I'm one of those crazy fools. I've been dragged across the river before, sputtering and gasping and left cold and exhausted on the other side. But now I know a better way. You can stay over there with the others, afraid of getting tangled in the weeds and drowning, but I can tell you some secrets about swimming by your own strength – secrets even the lifeguards don't know.

Sure it's chilly at first, but once you get used to it, the water's fine. Did you know how free and light you feel floating in the cool water, kicking your legs, stretching your arms and bending in ways you can't on land? And without the darn noisy motorboat, did you know the water makes a wonderful, soothing rippling sound? And when you swim alone, you swim however you want. There breaststroke is popular, or the sidestroke. The backstroke is slower, but you can look at the sky while you swim. In fact, you can invent your own stroke, something unheard of with a trained lifeguard. Go as fast or as slow as you want; there's no reason to hurry and get out of breath. You'll probably be tired by the time you reach the other side, and you'll be relieved to see the other shore, but you'll feel absolutely wonderful, triumphant, when you reach the shore by your own strength.

And pssst! Have you ever tried skinny-dipping in the moonlight with your lover? Incredible!

A Bit of Advice

One of the most awkward things to deal with in pregnancy is unsolicited advice, particularly with the first baby. Anybody who has ever had a baby knows more than you do. Everyone has been there, done that, and therefore an expert on which is the best way to give birth, and the best way to raise the baby. (Including me, of course — I'm just as annoying as everybody else is.)

"The epidural was wonderful," one says, "I didn't feel a thing!" Another tells how much the epidural hurt. "Take all the medicine they offer you, and you'll enjoy the birth more." "Take nothing - it's bad for the baby!" "Don't go to the hospital too soon or you will be subject to a lot of intervention." "Don't go to the hospital too late or you risk having the baby in the car."

It's so confusing you turn to books, and they are no better. This one says the episiotomy protects you from a tear, another says it can make a tear worse. One person says homebirth is wonderful another one says it is dangerous.

Who are you supposed to believe? Where do you go for advice? Who are the real experts? People with more schooling? More years of clinical practice?

One woman I know highly recommends her doctor for expert advice on everything from breastfeeding to toddler tantrums to how to get the baby to sleep through the night. Why, I wonder? Why does she think the doctor should know all the answers? He is trained in *medicine*, and his job is to treat disease with medicine. He's not supposed to be an expert on parenting. You'd probably get equally good advice from your mechanic.

Another woman I know gives a lot of weight to the medical advice from her friend who has worked in the hospital for many years. Why it matters, I don't know, because the friend works in the hospital as a *cleaning lady*!

Before I got my real job as a parent, I worked in a large psychiatric hospital. During my orientation and training program I learned many of the marriage counselors on staff were divorced. This was good, I was told, because they knew where marriage could go wrong, and their personal experience with a soured marriage could help struggling couples overcome their problems. I guess I started to smirk at this information, because my instructor abruptly wanted to know what I found so amusing.

"Why would I go to someone for marriage counseling," I asked, "Who doesn't know how to stay married themselves?" If they had learned what went wrong and were now happily married, then I would listen.

When I had my baby, I kept getting breastfeeding advice from people who were not able to breastfeed! Why would I want to listen to them? If, however she learned what had gone wrong and successfully nursed a second child, then I know I could learn a lot from her.

A clergyman offered me some parenting advice when he was visiting one day. He watched me making tea one-handed; handicapped by a fussy baby in my other arm, then respectfully informed me of how I was spoiling my child by carrying him. I was advised to leave him alone in his crib when I was doing important things, so the baby would learn there were more important things in life (like making tea) and baby would simply have to wait until the important things were done. That's what he did with his children, he said, and it worked. They certainly didn't get coddled, no sir. I considered his advice until later in the conversation when he happened to mention one of his sons was in jail and the other was a drug addict. *Not spoiled, but ruined*, I thought. I picked up my fussy baby, who was certainly one of the most important things in my life, and "spoiled" him some more.

Obstetricians, Family Physicians, Midwives

An important source of childbirth advice comes from childbirth books written by medical doctors. They contain helpful information from a medical perspective. I am very happy to live in a country where we have excellent, well-trained, and experienced doctors available. But for the woman wanting a birth free from unnecessary medical intervention, a medical doctor is not the person to ask for advice on unmedicated natural childbirth.

The general physician cannot help but see childbirth from the perspective he was taught. He was taught medicine. He practices medicine. He knows what drugs to use to induce labour and what drugs will relieve pain. His training focuses on pathology - abnormal childbirth - and how medicine can help pathological conditions.

An obstetrician specializes in obstetrical surgery. Through his training and experience with difficult births, he knows how to surgically deliver babies in problematic situations. Obstetrics, being a surgical specialty, can offer the labouring woman little beyond technological tools and pain medicines. The obstetrician cannot take the time to sit with the mother during a long labour. He checks on her progress frequently to make sure there are no pathological problems and then depends on the nurses to call him when birth is imminent.

The midwife, on the other hand, is an expert on normal deliveries. Her training and experience focus on the course of typical, problem-free births, of which doctors will agree, make up over ninety percent of all deliveries. Because of her vast experience with normal birth, the midwife quickly recognizes an abnormality, and will seek immediate medical attention if required. Therefore the midwife is better experienced in managing <u>natural</u> childbirth than a doctor is.

Taking Control

The midwife's job requires her to stay with the mother throughout the entire labour giving hands-on practical help: She has words of encouragement, helpful suggestions such as a change of position or a warm bath; and time — hours of time — spent with the mother throughout her labour. She rubs the sore back, massages the aching hips, and hugs the tearful frustration away in a woman-to-woman moment of connectedness. It's not the doctor's job nor is it even *appropriate* for a strange man to comfort a labouring woman in such a manner.

"There is no reason whatsoever for specialist obstetricians to be the health workers providing obstetrical care for normal healthy women," says Dr. Cynthia Carver[4]. Some women think they are better off with an obstetrician because he has the most years of education. But the obstetrician does not specialize in natural childbirth, and may actually have very little experience with a normal, natural, simple, unadulterated birth.

Asking a doctor if you'll need his medical assistance is like asking an insurance salesman if you need more insurance, like asking your Tupperware lady if you need more Tupperware, or the Filter Queen Salesman if you need a new vacuum cleaner. He wants your business.

The midwife considers the miracle of childbirth as normal, and leaves it alone unless there's trouble. The obstetrician normally sees childbirth as trouble; if he leaves it alone, it's a miracle.

Psychological Factors

No matter how many babies the doctor has caught, cut, or pulled out of women, a male doctor can never know what it <u>feels</u> like to give birth! Does it matter? Should it make any difference if we take a male perspective of a female function?

Well how do you think your husband would feel if most urologists were women? What if he had to go to a woman for his prostrate trouble or premature ejaculation? Would he feel comfortable in explaining his impotence? What if the female urologist considered his concerns about impotence irrelevant? We know a man would rather speak to another man about specifically male problems, yet why don't we consider the same logic regarding women's issues?

Does the doctor really understand what it means to a woman to discover a new life growing inside her body? Can he comprehend the secret communication between a mother and her unborn child — her response to the faint fluttering of movement when she first feels life; the rolling waves in her belly as the baby stretches, the sharp poke of elbows and heels under her ribs; the twisting jab caused by the turning of a little head near her bladder in the last weeks? Does he understand the fierce protectiveness a mother has for her child, even before it is born? Does he give any depth of meaning to the sexual expression of childbirth, and the effect it has on the couple as they complete their act of procreation this moment?

Does he care about the outpouring of love flooding from a woman's soul as she sees her child for the first time? Will he ever comprehend the joy of nourishing a new life after birth with the warm, sweet milk made from her body? Can he fully appreciate the pride and fulfillment a woman has watching her baby grow plump from her milk? Heck, if he's like most men, he probably doesn't even understand his own wife half the time; how's he ever going to understand you?

The Real Experts

Would you ask a beggar where you should invest your money? You wouldn't ask a fat person for the best weight-loss diet. In fact, if you want to lose weight, will it do any good to ask someone who has always been thin? Someone who knows what it's like to have a weight problem — and conquer it — could empathize with your problem better and encourage you along the way because of their own experience.

If you want to succeed, you look for successful people. And a person who has "been there" can give you advice based on experience.

Patricia Carter is one person who has "been there." She gave birth to seven of her babies at home, completely unassisted. While we might think she took a tremendous risk, we can certainly learn something from her success and experience with painless childbirth. You will read more about Mrs. Carter's experiences later.

In the 1950's when doctors were telling women they had "evolved" to the point they were no longer capable of breastfeeding their babies, seven nursing mothers got together with some friends and taught them they could indeed nurse if they wanted to with correct information, encouragement and support. La Leche League was founded by those seven women who learned the hard way how to successfully breastfeed their babies, and shared the information with others, mother-to-mother. These women, simply housewives and mothers who cared, helped take baby care and feeding out of the doctor's hands, and put it back in the mother's arms where it belonged.

While doctors were still insisting "Once a Cesarean, Always a Cesarean," and the rate of cesarean sections was climbing as high as fifty percent in some hospitals, two women researched the problem and wrote a book about it. *Silent Knife* by Nancy Wainer Cohen and

Lois J. Estner exposed the truth: VBAC is safer than repeat cesarean, and far too many c-sections are being done in the first place. *Silent Knife* is full of stories from women who have conquered the problems with information and ideas of what causes the problems and how to avoid them. Women who I met within the pages of this book gave me much better information on how to achieve VBAC than my skilled obstetrician did! Hundreds of women just like me, looked at the risks of VBAC vs. cesarean, and put the decision-making where it belongs, with the pregnant women.

A mainstream Canadian parenting magazine refused to publish a story about a beautiful homebirth, claiming it would be "controversial," and asked the writer to compose a story about the heroism in the Neonatal Intensive Care Unit. But the writer had a better idea. She quit working for a magazine which bowed to the demands of the powerful advertising companies, and on a small budget, started her own magazine. The *Compleat Mother* Magazine was born: bold, radical, and unashamed in proclaiming the raw beauty and profoundly emotional experiences of childbirth and breastfeeding, the way women truly experience it, both good and bad.

This Canadian publication is a treasure chest of mothering wisdom, empowering birth stories, and up-to-date reports on the medical studies related to pregnancy, birth, and breastfeeding. The *Compleat Mother* would prefer to remain a small-budget magazine than accept advertising money from those selling other products which undermine a woman's ability to meet her baby's needs by herself. Catherine Young, founder of the magazine, looked at the power and glory bestowed upon the doctor in the glossy magazines, and gave the might and power back to the woman giving birth, where it belongs.[i]

Don't Take It Lying Down!

My first suggestion or number one rule for making labour easier is this: STAY ON YOUR FEET.

In the hospital the first thing they do upon admission is issue you one of those ugly backless nightgown-things, and show you to a bed. But you are not like other patients – you don't have an illness and don't need treatment. But you are doing the important job of bringing forth a new life. STAY ON YOUR FEET, therefore, because you have a job to do.

STAY ON YOUR FEET and keep walking because sick, weak people are the ones who need to be in bed. Try to think of yourself as

[i] For online information go to www.compleatmother.com

a client, using a service, not a patient. Keep upright and keep walking, so you feel freedom to move and not confinement.

STAY ON YOUR FEET, because it raises you up to eye level, where you won't be looked down upon.

STAY ON YOUR FEET like a capable, *healthy* person, confident and in control.

STAY ON YOUR FEET, because gravity helps the baby to move down, pressing on the cervix, shortening your labour.

STAY ON YOUR FEET because there is less pain when the weight of the uterus is not pressing on your back.

STAY ON YOUR FEET, because when you lie down, the very bed you lie upon offers resistance to your pelvis, which is doing its best to open up for the baby.

STAY ON YOUR FEET, walking, walking, walking through the contractions, rocking, rocking, easing your baby lower and deeper into the birth canal.

STAY ON YOUR FEET so the doctors and nurses can't keep invading your body with their painful vaginal exams. They'll have to ask you to get onto the bed, which gives you the option of saying no! If you STAY ON YOUR FEET they'll only be able to do things when *you're* ready to let them. If you STAY ON YOUR FEET, you can look them in the eye, say no, and walk away.

STAY ON YOUR FEET, walking, refusing a lot of unnecessary vaginal exams, until you realize your body is pushing.

How long can you stay on your feet? Well, if you like, you can push while you are standing, or you can go down into a squat, to deliver your baby. <u>You don't need to lie down to have a baby</u>!

Does it surprise you to know the 'lying on your back, legs in stirrups' position is the WORST position for giving birth? It's bad for the mother and bad for the baby, but the doctor needs you on your back because it makes *his* job easier.

Hey, wait a minute! Whose comfort *should* be of concern? Whose job *should* we make easier? There are three very important players in this birth scene: There's the woman in labour: in pain, struggling to give birth to a new life, pushing with all her might to get a human being through her pelvic bones. No, we won't worry about her comfort, except to give her some drugs. There's the baby, who may be oxygen-deprived if the mother lies on her back, causing fetal distress. No, don't worry about the baby, we'll resuscitate if we have to. Then there's the doctor, who is being paid—*well* paid—to catch the baby. Let's make sure *he's* comfortable! Does this make sense?

Staying on your feet and walking is helpful not only because it makes good sense physiologically to work *with* gravity instead of *against* it; more importantly, it has to do with how it makes you feel about yourself. A simple thing like staying out of bed makes you feel more capable, confident, and ready to take on the challenge! Lying in bed makes you feel more like a weak, sick person; like a little girl, dependent upon others instead of an adult doing the most grown-up, womanly thing she can do. Not to mention how lying on your back forces your uterus to push a baby out *upwards,* over the tailbone! In an upright position, the baby comes out faster, pushing is more effective, and the baby is not pressing against your back.

Pick up any book on childbirth and look for the drawings where they show the birth complete with an "inside view." It shows the mother on her back. Now turn the book sideways, and note the angle at which the baby emerges when the mother is upright. Which would be easier?

The doctor prefers you on your back because it makes it easier for him:

- to do an episiotomy — which he won't need to do if you are upright, because the weight of the baby is not resting on the perineum;
- to use forceps to pull the baby out — which he won't need to do if you are upright because you will be able to push more effectively;
- to get the baby out faster — which he won't need to do because the baby won't be distressed from the lack of oxygen it would experience if you were on your back;
- to keep close watch on the mother's blood pressure — which isn't as much of a concern when she is upright and in control and not exhausting herself from ineffective pushing, or getting dizzy from the weight of the baby pressing on the major blood vessels as she lies on her back

It may not seem like a big deal, pushing the baby upwards, but think how hard it is to work against gravity for easy things. Yesterday I was hammering a nail up above my head, and I found it hard pushing a 16-ounce hammer up into the air each time; much more tiring than nailing something lower.

In fact, if your doctor thinks it doesn't make much difference pushing against gravity, agree with him: since *he* says it's no big deal, let *him* work against gravity. He can catch the baby from beneath while you give birth comfortably low; squatting, kneeling, or reclined in an armchair.

Whatever Works

Now, before you go out and buy some sturdy hiking boots for your labour kit, I can't finish this section without reminding you that walking was what worked for *me*. I was with a friend who was in labour a while back, and she was perfectly content to lie on her couch in labour. She looked so relaxed, stretched out on her side, she reminded me of a mother cat contentedly waiting for her litter to be born. "I just hope it's soon," she purred.

Some women like to spend their entire labour rocking in their favorite rocking chair. Others like to sit on the toilet, which makes good sense, because the toilet is one place where we are accustomed to relaxing the muscles of the pelvic floor.

Patricia Carter, who had seven babies unassisted, believes the key to an easy birth is in relaxation of the pelvic floor.

> [B]y getting the weight off the pelvic floor ahead of time one helps to secure softening and relaxation of the muscles in the birth canal, which must relax and enlarge for egress of the child. I do not mean that I lie down like a recumbent statue during all the first stage, but in general I do try to keep the weight off the bottom."[5]

She preferred to rest while in labour, writing letters, doing her nails or putting on make-up, only getting up for short periods.

> The laziest and most relaxed figures I can imagine are those of the Ancients at their banquets, half recumbent upon their low couches, the beautiful Grecian figures portraying ease and comfort with every line the artist made. I try to emulate them, and pillow my couch likewise. This satisfies instinct better than a bed. Nature wants no women prone on their backs in a helpless position at such a time, but free to lean on their elbows. To be relaxed, but not helpless.[6]

The trick is then, to do what *your body* tells you to do. Listen to your body. What worked for somebody else might not work for you. One person feels better relaxing in bed; another likes to rock in a rocking chair. Many women like to stay in the bathtub. I personally found it more painful to sit still, agony to lie in bed, and sheer torture to be told I had to stay there.

Many women are discovering the benefit of labouring in the tub. A British midwife reports:

> "Beds are useless things in labour. Women labour safely in privacy, darkness and comfortable positions on soft flooring.
>
> "We base our practice on homebirths and find women normally give birth standing up or on all fours.
>
> "Lots of women have laboured in the bath over centuries. Pools give a woman privacy — it's her space; it helps a woman control pain. In that environment she releases endorphins enormously and her baby is suffused with endorphins.
>
> "We don't get in the pool. For one thing there is often blood and poo floating in it, for another it is the place for her and her partner and perhaps young children.

> "Women in waterbirth are more assertive and less likely to listen to their midwife." Frequently the men say it's a good idea to listen to the baby's heart rate, and the water-laboring moms will say 'not now' and swim off.[7]

Your Birthday Suit

If you are going to be up and walking around throughout labour, make sure you wear something which makes you feel pretty! Most women care a lot about how they dress, and some will plan weeks in advance what they are going to wear for a special occasion. What occasion could be more special than the birth of your baby? On a day as unique and wonderful as your baby's birthday, why be denied the same exciting anticipation in choosing the perfect outfit? Nobody likes to parade around in one of those ugly Hospital Patient Uniforms, your butt exposed for the world to see!

It's bad enough to wear a Hospital Patient Uniform when you are sick, like the other inmates, but a woman in labour is not sick, so why not pick out something different for yourself? You might like something colourful and cheery, in sharp contrast to the usual hospital colours. Make this day your celebration by picking something fabulous to wear! One friend of mine chose an extra-long shirt with buttons all down the front which she could undo if she felt too warm, also for easy access to breastfeeding. Some women like to wear a comfortable T-shirt, or a loose, flowing dress. Others like to feel sexy, and choose something lacy and silky. Why not? Feeling sexy gets the right hormones pumping through your body. Besides, those high-heeled pumps will make squatting easier!

If you are any good at sewing, you might want to make your own special birthing gown. In fact, there's a great new business opportunity: custom-designed birthing wear! Start your own business and get rich quicker than you can say *epidural*!

Don't be too surprised if the hospital staff gives you a hard time over you wearing your custom-made Birth Day Suit. Be pleasant about it, but firm. They just aren't used to the idea. I had a bit of an argument with the nurse when I pulled out my pretty lace nightgown I had planned to wear for my baby's birth. She tried to convince me not to wear it because it might get soiled. I tried to explain, between contractions, why I didn't care if it got soiled. I bought it specifically for this messy occasion! What difference should it make to them, what I wear? Are they afraid they'd have to wash it if it becomes soiled? No, my husband or I would wash it (or throw it away). Worried it might get lost? So what? Are they afraid of germs? I feel much safer with my own friendly germs from home than in their

Hospital Patient Uniform worn by the last guy recovering from Flesh-Eating Disease.

One underlying reason they don't want you wearing your own clothing is because wearing a Hospital Patient Uniform puts you in your place. "Uniform" means plain, unvaried, just like the rest. They don't want you autonomous. They want you compliant.

I had purchased the silky nightgown just for my special occasion. If it got soiled, so what? I picked it out with as much happy anticipation as shopping for my wedding gown. On my wedding day, I fully expected my gown might get dirty. It might get wine or food spilled on it, or might get sweaty from dancing, but nothing would stop me from wearing it!

My nightgown did get a little blood on it, which rinsed out as good as new. I considered it my "lucky" nightgown and wore it for my next birth. (My wedding gown got dirty too. I stepped in dog poop.)

One final thought about your birth day suit: no matter what you choose to wear, you can and you may change your mind at any time. Some women find themselves feeling so "earthy" during labour, they suddenly rip their clothes off and squat down to give birth naked and sweaty and grunting like a caveman.

When Push Comes to Shove

The sign on the delivery room door swings inward. *Push*, it says. How appropriate.

The second stage of labour has finally arrived, and the doctor coaches you on when and how to push. It's exhausting and exhilarating at the same time. With each push you can feel the baby move down a little farther. As the baby's head appears everyone gets more excited and yells all the more, PUSH! PUSH! And you, propped up on pillows, your husband supporting your shoulders, yell back, "I AM pushing, DAMMIT!"

Why in the world do they assume that unless a team of medical staff scream at the mother, the baby would just stay inside the birth canal forever?

Wait a minute, you see the doctor get the forceps! You glance back at the delivery room door again. *Pull*, it says on this side! Yikes!

A recent study showed that when women were *not* coached when and how to push, as is the usual practice, their pushing contractions were handled differently: some strong pushes, some gentle pushes, and sometimes not pushing at all during contractions[8]. This makes perfect sense! It's been called *listening to your body*, and it's nothing new. Perhaps her body says, *"Time to get started - push hard! Again! Hold on — go easy now, easy, while the baby's head gets past the pubic bone. Okay, now give a good one to get the body down farther... ease off now, we're getting close to the perineum... easy does it, the shoulder is coming round the bend... there! Okay, another big one. Careful now, let those tissues stretch..."*

When nurses holler at the woman to tell her when to push — based on what they see going on from the outside – it tells the woman she cannot trust her own body to know what to do. Her subconscious mind believes she can't do it without their help; and she certainly can't trust her own instinctive response. *Listen to US*, the message is, *don't trust yourself. Don't listen to your body*. Believe me, your body probably has a better idea of what's going on inside than all the pairs of eyes staring so rudely between your legs.

When I had my second homebirth, I was very aware of what was going on as I started pushing. Feeling a slight tightness on the perineum, I'd instinctively quit pushing to pant lightly until the sensation eased. "Stop pushing," the doctor said. As the skin on the perineum adjusted to the stretching, I'd gently push for a few seconds, only to hear the doctor to tell me, "Now, push!" but by then I was panting again, having felt the tightening and tension in the perineum. The doctor's coaching was distracting: I would be aware of my body, responding to its cues, and then the doctor's instruction would interrupt my concentration, confusing me as to what I should be doing. Should I keep doing what feels right, what seems to be working? Or listen to him, the expert?

After a couple of minutes the doctor realized I was already *doing* what he was trying to coach me to do! He stopped mid-sentence and shrugged to my husband, "I guess she already knows!" Then he sat quietly and let me continue, and I very gently, very quietly birthed my 10 lb. 3 oz baby girl without a bruise or stitch or struggle.

In such a highly aware state, concentrating, "listening" to my body I could tell the exact position my baby was in. I felt her ears being born, her nose, her chin. Incredible!

The birth also had a surprising impact on the doctor, who was not my regular family doctor; but he was the only one in this part of Ontario who would come to a home birth. On my daughter's first birthday he phoned me to tell me he had not forgotten what an incredible birth it was. Some births are so special, he said, they rest in his memory forever. Mine was one of them, and he just wanted me to know.

I was surprised. *My* baby's birth? Imprinted on the doctor's mind forever? What was so great about another birth of another baby to a doctor who's delivered hundreds? Had he not remembered how I swore at him when I was in transition?

I called his office back and made an appointment to see him the next day. I brought him a big slice of my daughter's birthday cake and we had a nice little chat while he did a quick checkup on the baby to satisfy the insurance people. And yes, he remembered how I swore at him.

At my next birth, the doctor missed the birth by a half-hour. With nobody to tell me how far dilated I was, and whether or not it was "time" to push, I simply did what came naturally. I was standing up when I felt the baby slip down into the birth canal. Instinctively, I sat down on the floor and leaned back against the side of the bed, opened my legs, and simply *let the baby come out.* There really wasn't any pushing.

Perhaps I was fully dilated for an hour before the baby was born. If the doctor had been there to check me and tell me to push an hour earlier, it may have taken several minutes of straining. Does it not make sense to let our bodies push when we are ready, rather than when someone tells us we should?

Patricia Carter, in her description of unattended birth, said she simply relaxed on her couch in the privacy of her bedroom, and trusted her body to do its job all by itself - the less interference, the better.

> ... everything will go along smoothly, painlessly, and at the exact instant the door is open, up will rise the old fundus, like a jet ready for the takeoff. One extra powerful squeeze and it starts the baby down that bony passage with such a good strong takeoff, the baby won't stop till it's thru the tunnel, rounds that bend, hits street level, so to speak, and slides Whee! out into the light of day.[9]

Too Pooped?

As much as I hate to compare childbirth to having a bowel movement, there are some obvious comparisons. Many people, who have no problem at home, require laxatives when they are in the hospital. For some, just being away from home on vacation is enough to cause constipation. Some people just can't relax the same unless they have their own bathroom.

Did you ever try to use a bedpan? As much as it is awkward and uncomfortable, comfort is not the only concern. What's really hard to overcome is having other patients in the room who can hear what you are doing! (If they don't hear you they may get wind of it another way.) And the nurse is hanging around waiting to collect your deposit, carry it somewhere, even inspect it before she flushes it and records it in her notes. What if a doctor, a resident, an intern and two nurses had to observe the whole thing?

"Push! Push!" they would all yell in unison. Your husband would hold your hand to support you and encourage you as you strain to push when there is no urge to do so. The doctor tells you when to stop pushing so as to avoid the risk of hemorrhoids and anal fissures. In fact, he may even perform a rectumotomy! "It's just a little cut," he says.

Forgive me for this disgusting comparison. Childbirth is not a function of elimination; it is part of our sexual function. Sheila Kitzinger, social anthropologist and author of several books on childbirth stated,

> Think what it would be like if someone stood by you, telling you to "Empty your bowels, hurry up, get it done in ten minutes." Think about if someone stood over you saying, "Have that orgasm, you've got 15 minutes or we'll do it for you." It's the same when a doctor or a nurse tells us to "Dilate, and Push, Push, Push." The challenge to us is to rediscover the sexual joy and energy to return birth to normal expression.[10]

Private events should happen in privacy. Giving birth uses our private parts, and it's embarrassing to have others watch.

"But we are logical, intelligent creatures," you reason, "We rise above such embarrassment and deliver our babies into the hands of the doctor because we understand he is the person who best can ensure the safety of both mother and child." Of course you can, if you have to. But we are talking about giving birth *easily,* and birth is easier if you are not inhibited.

My point is that pushing a baby out comes as <u>easily</u> and instinctively as a bowel movement, quickly and smoothly, if you push when *you* are ready, *not when the doctor thinks you are ready.* Instead of learning to listen to your body, we have been trained too much to rely on the doctor or midwife telling us when and how to do it. We get mixed up and confused by what they tell us and what we feel. We don't know who to listen to, and it causes tension. I *don't feel like pushing, but the doctor says I must. I must be wrong. I can't listen to what my body says. I can't trust it to do the right thing.*

I've often wondered why we actually have to deliver into the doctor's hands, anyway. Is there some magic in those hands? How many women are forced into panting to keep from pushing, holding off the birth for the doctor's arrival? Poor dad has been with her for hours, rubbing her back, encouraging her, and loving her, helping her through each contraction. The doctor arrives at the last minute, catches the baby, and gets all the credit. The dad should rightfully get the credit.

Why couldn't we deliver into our husband's hands? In fact, why couldn't they allow couples their privacy in the labour and delivery room, knowing they could call for help from the staff if needed? If help is not needed, why bother the doctor?

It's really a shame to waste a skilled obstetrician's time and expertise on a normal healthy delivery. What a waste of his years of training and experience to sit around watching a healthy mother giving birth to a healthy baby when it's not required. It's like using a blowtorch to light a candle: it's just not necessary.

Your Poor Pussy

Women should be given the same respect we give to our cats and dogs when they are birthing. When your cat is having kittens, how many times do you take her to the vet during her gestation to make sure she is growing properly? How many blood tests do you subject her to? Does the vet restrict her diet? Does he measure her bones to insure her pelvis is adequate?

When you notice she is having contractions would you rush her off to the vet? We all know the vet's office makes animals nervous, likely because they associate it with needles. Not only would your pussycat be more nervous and uptight in the vet's office, suppose the vet put her on her back to see the kittens emerge better. Suppose he puts an IV in her, just in case, and keeps disturbing her with uncomfortable examinations. He puts a strap on her belly to monitor her contractions. Poor pussy has to deal with increasingly intense contractions as well as all these strange, frightening experiences. How do you think it would affect her performance? Do you think she'd be able to have her kittens in the vet's office as easily as she would in the quiet dark corner of your closet? In her own home, she simply seeks a quiet spot surrounded by the usual sounds and familiar smells which give her comfort in her pain until she finally gives birth on your best sweater.

It's The Thought That Counts:
The Power of Positive Thinking, Mind over Matter, Visualization and stuff

If you want a positive outcome, you have to think positive. Don't ask me how it works, but it does. Don't be like the fellow in the book by Dr. Seuss who would not, could not eat green eggs and ham.

I cannot do this without drugs, I cannot birth with only hugs.

I cannot birth unless in bed, the doc said I would lose my head.

I cannot labour if I walk, it can't be done. Just ask the doc!

Fill your mind with the wrong kind of images and you will influence the outcome of your birth.

I don't want to get fat so I won't think about chocolate cake. I refuse to think about chocolate cake. I will not think of sweet dark chocolate cake. Dark chocolate cake with the creamy icing...I will not think of how good the rich chocolate cake would taste right now. I will not think about how I'm a little hungry. And I worked all day and come to think of it — I deserve a piece of cake!

You must fill your mind with positive thoughts and images, and you will help it become a reality:

I am healthy and strong. I am eating well and taking good care of myself. I am a growing a healthy baby. I'm strong and patient and have great endurance.

(For VBAC: I'm going to have a vaginal birth this time. It's going to be an exciting experience! My scar has healed completely, just like any other cut I've ever had. My body is designed for giving birth, especially one as healthy as mine. I eat well and take care of myself, and I'm healthy and strong.)

Picture yourself giving birth with joy and confidence. When you get fearful — and you will because you're normal — force yourself to focus on the positive. For example suppose you hear a birth horror story from someone describing the awful things going wrong at her birth. You wonder: *What if it happens to me?* Don't run from your fears, worrying *Oh I hope it doesn't happen to me!* Face the fear instead. Imagine yourself in the same situation, but imagine yourself in control and making wise, informed decisions and actively seeking alternative solutions to the problems.

Only a few weeks away from delivering my fourth baby, there was a show about births on the TV. I couldn't bear to watch it because of the moaning and wailing of one of the women. (Another good reason not to have your baby in the hospital: the wails and screams of other labouring women.) I taped the show though, to watch one afternoon when the children were napping and I could allow myself a good cry. And cry I did, a box of tissues on my lap, empathizing with the wailing woman in the film, knowing the weeping woman would soon be me. Having faced the dragon, I was no longer afraid of it. I knew I could handle it. *I'm tough enough*, I told myself. It really wasn't so scary after all.

Some people wail and moan as a way of dealing with pain, others suffer in silence. Some whine. What do you feel like doing? How do you handle pain when you stub your toe for instance? Do you scream, cry, run for an aspirin, or take a deep breath, and realize it will stop throbbing in a couple of minutes.

Imagine the kind of birth you want to have. Dream about your ideal birth? Picture yourself in labour, dealing with the pain in constructive ways. This is not so you can make it happen exactly as in your dream, because it's not realistic; but it helps to imagine different scenarios, different ways you can make a great birth happen no matter what the situation.

Dream and imagine as you might with your sex life, fantasizing freely about the perfect birth, even if not a realistic scenario. Share your birth dreams with your husband; so he gets an idea of what you would like and will better be able to help fulfill your wishes, both in bed and in the delivery room. That's his job.

One woman pictures herself giving birth at the beach, the waves crashing on the shore in rhythm with the power of her contractions. Another imagines herself giving birth in a quiet cabin in the woods by a crackling fire, or on a mountain, with the scent of pine trees and the sound of birds singing all about. What this exercise does is help replace the media image of painful screaming childbirth with a more pleasant one.

When in labour, visualize with each contraction what is happening inside you. Imagine your cervix is opening and stretching more and more with each contraction. Visualize the baby, moving down lower and deeper with each squeeze of the fundus. Imagine what it feels like for the baby inside, moving, slowly, down, down.

Consumer Demand

If we want to make changes in the way childbirth is handled, we have to assert ourselves and have the guts to follow through. Take heart: we have made tremendous changes in the medical system already. Let's not give up yet.

Dr. Cynthia Carver, well-known columnist for Chatelaine Magazine, says,

> "It suited doctors to a "T" to have encouraged a great mystique around birth, and to have everything about it totally in their control. They were accountable to no one; no one knew enough to complain or criticize or even to shout "negligence" or "malpractice." *The situation has now changed dramatically in some hospitals due almost entirely to the efforts of women patients, childbirth educators and men who cared...*" [11] [Italics added]

She comments on the changes she has seen in the delivery room as a result of consumer (that's YOU!) demands:

> There were studies showing that shaving pubic hair increased rather than decreased infection; that walking around instead of lying in bed improved labour; that women accompanied by a coach progressed better than those left to labour alone; that bonding with infants improved if they were held and cuddled by parents in the delivery room; that anesthetics and analgesics caused the babies to be less alert at birth; that nursing newborns frequently, on demand, permitted better milk production and faster growth; that breast milk was better for infants than formula. For years doctors managed not

> to research any of these issues, and when some statistics began coming in, they pooh-poohed or ignored them.
>
> After a while, much of the "factual" information I was taught as a student began to disappear from lectures: that forceps births were good for mother and infant because they shortened the pushing stage of labour, thus sparing the baby's head and the mother's perineum; that shaving pubic hair prevented infection; that babies must be given water or formula in the nursery to prevent dehydration; that after birth babies must be kept in isolation for twenty-four hours in the nursery to prevent infection any many, many other "scientific" wisdoms.[12]

Remember, doctors were perfectly happy with things the way they were. It was women who made these changes come about in the delivery room. Women like you and me and our sisters and mothers before us.

Isn't it nice to know science has finally proven true the things mothers have instinctively known all along? Isn't it nice to know, after generations of women were left with an aching emptiness in their arms, a desperate longing for their babies, and a feeling of detachment after giving birth, that science has declared mothers bond better with their babies when they are allowed to *see* them? Isn't it nice to know studies have proven women labour better when accompanied by someone who cares about them, rather than alone or with strangers? Isn't it nice to know the milk we women produce in our own bodies is far superior to any of the man-made formulas doctors have been telling us to spend our money on for years? Isn't it annoying to realize whatever the inherent female impulse drove women to do, it was ignored as irrelevant to the authority of science, until the almighty name of science proved women were right after all? Isn't it infuriating how we were presumed guilty until proven innocent?

With all due respect for science, my first reaction to the results of these types of studies is usually, "Well, duh!" One typical study which was mentioned in all the parenting magazines discovered babies cried less when they were held more. Well, duh! Ask any five-year-old if she thinks her new baby brother will be happier in his crib or on Mommy's lap. Do they have to spend thousands of dollars on a study to prove something obvious? Why didn't they *just ask?*

"Mrs. Smith, would you feel more comfortable if the man you love, the father of this child, the one who shares your bed, your home, and your life, also shared the birth of his child? Or would you rather we send him off to get drunk while you spend the next several hours alone? Would you rather walk around in labour, and move according to your comfort level, or shall we drug you senseless and restrain you in bed?"

Preparing the Body

One wise woman told me giving birth easily is 90% mental attitude. I think she's right. They say good sex is 90% attitude, too. Nevertheless, there are a few ideas which may be of help, none of which I can guarantee have been scientifically proven.

1. Eat well. Everything going into your mouth should be something good for you. Food expert Adelle Davis[13] suggested the following nutrients might help ease suffering in labour:
   - Calcium has been known to decrease sensitivity to pain.
   - laboratory studies showed prolonged labour in zinc-deficient rats
   - protein deficiency in animals can cause weakness, late and difficult deliveries
   - low magnesium in the blood can lead to weak muscles
   - potassium is essential to muscular contractions so it might be wise to increase in last few weeks of pregnancy
   - Vitamin E keeps vaginal tissues elastic, lessens likelihood of stretch marks and phlebitis, decreases need for oxygen. Lack of vitamin in animals causes degeneration of skeletal muscles
   - Vitamin C also keeps elasticity in vaginal tissues and can prevent premature rupture of the membranes.
2. Nap every day. You're sleeping for two. Even twenty minutes can be surprisingly refreshing. Not only the last trimester when you are carrying extra weight around, but even in the first trimester when you don't even look pregnant yet, your body is at work growing the baby's major organs and brain cells, and needs rest. <u>All mammals</u> nap, though in our culture we often consider it a sign of laziness. Too bad. You need more rest; period.
3. Raspberry Leaf Tea is one of the best known herbs for women. Ancient wise-woman wisdom, your doctor likely won't know about, or might consider it dangerous (some herbs are). Raspberry Leaf is tea is good for all female conditions, to ease childbirth, menstrual cramps and mood swings. Make your own or get it from the health food store or mail-order from *Compleat Mother* magazine. Hot or cold, drink it throughout your pregnancy, and more in the last weeks. Drink it in labour. Add honey if you don't like the taste.
4. At some health food stores you can get a five-week herbal formula to take the last five weeks of pregnancy. The herbs are said to soften the cervix, increase Braxton-Hicks contractions and reduce the bruised feeling after birth.

5. Chiropractic treatments can help you feel well-adjusted when the pregnant belly throws you out of alignment, and an out-of alignment pelvis can lead to a longer, more painful labour.
6. Orgasm tones the uterus. You figure it out. Keep fit and have fun.

CHAPTER 3

The Hard Way

> Doctors are men who prescribe medicines of which they know little, to cure diseases of which they know less, in human beings of whom they know nothing.
>
> -Voltaire

My great round belly protruding in front of me, I slouched down low in my favourite armchair until my bottom was even with the edge of the seat. *This would be a comfortable position for giving birth*, I thought.

"I'll go to the hospital for this baby, for our first," I said to my husband, "But I want to have the next baby at home."

"We'll see," was his non-committal reply. Bert knew I was determined to have this baby "natural" — without any medication. Together we went to not one, but two complete sets of prenatal classes; I was so hungry for information on how to do this.

First we signed up for the classes offered by the Public Health Department where we learned all about normal discomforts of pregnancy and how to deal with them; how to eat a well-balanced diet; and what to expect when we went into labour. Frankly I found these classes dull, lacking any new information beyond what one could read in any good childbirth book. An avid reader, I had already read every book on childbirth I could find in the public library. Since I wanted a natural, drug-free birth, I needed to find out how to do it... from someone who had *done* it.

The Pre-natal teacher — a nurse and mother of two — had never experienced an unmedicated birth. She taught us how we were supposed to breathe when we were in labour to help us remain in control. It was important to always stay In Control. Meaning, we were to be quiet. Making any noise was considered a lack of Control or a failure to follow the rules of breathing in order to handle the labour correctly. Better to have an epidural than to lose Control.

"Hhhooo.... Hhhooo...." We all practiced the breathing method to be used at four centimetres dilation. We diligently practiced the different levels of breathing to be used at the different stages of labour, and our husbands would pinch our legs during the breathing exercises to prove the breathing methods did indeed help distract us from pain.

"When you reach transition," the teacher instructed, "You should breathe like this, 'Hee-Hee-Hee...' But don't worry about it," she added, "Because you will have your epidural by then." I was the *only one* in the class who was not planning on having an epidural!

Disappointed by the lack of helpful information the Public Health Classes had given us, I signed up for some classes offered by an independent childbirth education organization. These classes were held in private homes while toddlers and older children scampered about. They were taught by mothers who had themselves given birth using these breathing methods and relaxation techniques. Someone who had *done* it!

How I loved hearing the teacher talk about her birth experiences. She was one of the few people I had ever met who had given birth without any drugs! I was impressed. Isn't awake and aware the way it should be? I couldn't imagine why women wouldn't want to be awake and aware and fully participating in the birth of their child, even if it was painful. Aren't you supposed to get over it quickly, forgetting the pain?

The Family Doctor

My doctor, on the other hand, didn't agree with my ideas for childbirth. Each visit I was beginning to feel more and more frustrated by his answers to my questions. I was irritated by his attitude, though at first I couldn't figure out why.

Dr. K. had been my family doctor since I was a baby. In fact, he delivered me. My mother and his wife had been friends, and so when my mother went to the hospital to give birth to me in 1959, she got a special privilege: she didn't have to have her hands tied down in the delivery room!

Dr. K had a small office of birch paneling which always smelled to me of antiseptic and illness. As I grew up I learned to ignore the butterflies-in-my-stomach feeling I would get every time I recognized the smell upon entering his office. It was truly a family practice: all my cousins; aunts and uncles in the area went to Dr. K.

The Hard Way

I had been married four years when I went smiling into Dr. K's office with my morning urine sample in a jam jar, declaring proudly, "I think I'm pregnant!"

"Do you want an abortion?" he asked, popping one of his scotch mints into his mouth.

My jaw dropped. "I - I'm married!" I stammered. He knew I was married, because he had the privilege of giving me my very first embarrassing internal exam, just before my wedding.

"It doesn't matter. Sometimes it's just not the right time." He leaned forward, tilted his head back, and peered through his bifocals. "So, you want this baby?"

"Of course I do!" I was shocked and hurt. Could he not see how happy I was when I came in?

"OK," he shrugged, "Hop up on the scales, then."

When I announced to my mother she was soon to become a grandmother, I told her how upset I was by his remark. She reminded me the doctor was only doing his job. Still, I thought it was callous.

On my next visit, when I told the doctor I wanted to have this baby "natural," he pooh-poohed the idea. He seemed to think natural childbirth was a silly notion, a crazy fad. He'd delivered a lot of babies over the years, he said, and most women can't manage very well without help. He'd given my own mother gas, he reminded me. Why would I think I could handle it if she couldn't?

"Animals," he informed me, "know instinctively how to give birth. But women don't. They need to be told."

Dr. K said only on rare occasions would he would allow a mother to give birth without drugs. Usually it was only if a woman was "tough" and had proven her ability to handle it with previous births. (I wondered how she could have had a previous birth without drugs, if he drugged all women for all births.) I simply didn't have what it takes, he said.

"You think you could handle a delivery without drugs?" he asked, jabbing the syringe into my vein for a blood test, "Look at you, how you flinch over a little needle!" I imagined childbirth hurt much more than a needle, but doubted if you could compare the two.

Women need to be told how to give birth. His comment stayed on my mind. Women need to be told how to give birth—by men? *Male* doctors, who have never given birth, are the only ones who know how to do it? *Male* doctors are the only ones qualified to direct the female act of childbirth? Huh? And if dumb animals can do it instinctively, why can't humans? Don't we have some animal instinct too?

The Last Straw

On my fifth monthly prenatal visit I brought up the subject of breastfeeding. Having read every book in the local library on childbirth by this time, I was moving onto the topics of breastfeeding and baby care. I knew breastfeeding was definitely the best choice. From The Womanly Art of Breastfeeding, I learned that immediate breastfeeding would help my uterus to contract, lowering the risk of hemorrhage; that in the first hour after delivery, the baby would be alert and eager to nurse; that while there would be no milk at first, the baby would be getting *colostrum*, a fluid rich in nutrients and important immune factors that would protect the baby from illness. Wow, all those benefits just from doing what nature intended!

I knew this had to be discussed ahead of time, not argued about at the time of delivery. When I told the doctor I would like to breastfeed as soon as the baby was born, he mumbled something about breastfeeding being a good choice for babies.

"But I mean right away," I clarified, "Right on the delivery table, as soon as the baby is born." Dr. K sighed loudly. It appeared as if I was making an unreasonable demand.

"I don't see what you need to do *that* for," he sniffed. "What's the point? You'll have plenty of time for *that* later. Besides, it doesn't do the baby any good, because there's no milk yet. It doesn't do you any good — well, it might make you *feel* good — but it just means we have to move all the sterile drapes and everyone will be too busy at the time."

I didn't pursue the matter any more. I didn't know what to say. I was astonished. He didn't know, he *really didn't know*, of the benefits of breastfeeding immediately after delivery! I was shocked! I thought doctors knew everything about the body, about childbirth, and about the health benefits of breastfeeding. I thought they were kept up-to-date on the latest research.

Besides, what's the big deal about moving a couple of sterile sheets to help a new mother cuddle and nurse her brand new baby? Isn't it their job?

After I dressed, I brought up another subject the doctor had never discussed with me: nutrition. The only thing he had said so far was not to gain more than 15 pounds.

"You're overweight to begin with," he had said, "Otherwise I'd let you gain up to twenty."

"Why? What will happen if I gain more?"

He leaned forward and peered at me over his bifocals. "You want your child to have a *fat* mother?"

On the chart he filled out during each visit I noticed there was a place to record the discussion of the mother's diet. I was five months along, and since he had not yet brought the subject of nutrition up, I did.

"Didn't I give you iron pills yet?" He asked, reaching for his prescription pad.

"Iron pills? Am I anemic?"

"No, but I'll give you some just in case."

"But I thought we are supposed to get all the vitamins we need from a well-balanced diet. How much iron do I need? Can't I get what I need by eating properly?"

"No, you can't. Just take one of these a day. Let me know if they make you constipated and I'll give you something to keep your bowels loose." He held out the prescription for me, but I didn't take it from him. I sat with my arms crossed, took a deep breath, and repeated myself.

"Tell me how much iron I need, and I will get it from food."

"You can't possibly get it from food. Everybody needs a prescription. I should have given it to you before."

"You mean to tell me a normal healthy pregnant woman cannot possibly get the vitamins she needs from a normal diet?"

"Right. One a day. Let me know if you get too constipated," he said, pushing the prescription at me, ending our discussion of nutrition.

Insulted, I snatched the paper from his hand. Eating well, it seemed, was not of any importance, but restricting weight gain and taking high, constipating doses of iron was. It didn't make sense to me how a normal condition like pregnancy should require a prescription. How would our species have survived if this were true?

It was unsettling to question Dr. K's authority, a man for whom I always had the greatest respect. He was the only doctor I ever had, and my whole family went to him, respected him, and liked him. Who was I to question this knowledgeable man, who had delivered probably hundreds of babies? And yet, I was becoming increasingly frustrated with his manner, and the condescending way he spoke to me. Why did I always leave there feeling like a naughty little girl?

With his patronizing attitude, lack of respect — even ridicule — of the things I wanted for the birth of my baby it was doubtful he would even let me attempt, let alone be supportive of, a natural childbirth. I only wanted some choice in things that were important to me but Dr. K would not allow any discussion. He was the boss. I didn't want to be treated like a little girl who "needed to be told." I was a grown woman, doing a grown-up thing. Maybe that was the problem: perhaps since Dr. K had known me since babyhood, he still saw me as a little girl. I guess it wasn't his fault; it was just time for me to grow up and move away.

Crushing the prescription into a ball, I tossed it back toward the office over my shoulder as I left the waiting room. I never went back.

In Doc We Trust

The Childbirth Education teacher gave me a list of doctors who were known to be supportive of natural childbirth. I picked one — based only on his convenient location (stupid me) — and made an appointment.

The new Dr.'s office was in a modern building shared by several health professionals with one central waiting room for all patients. It was very different having a new doctor for the first time in my life. I wrongly assumed all doctors handled pregnancy the same way in a standard prenatal visit and was therefore surprised to find Dr. S so different from Dr. K. Whereas Dr. K had taken blood tests every month, Dr. S said it wasn't necessary. However, Doctor S believed in doing a vaginal exam at each and every visit. Dr. S had several examining rooms on the go at once, where his patients would be ready and waiting for their appointment in their open-at-the-back hospital-type gowns. (It occurred to me later - I never actually spoke to Dr. S until I was already undressed.)

Dr. S was supportive of natural childbirth, and he actually encouraged breastfeeding. But oh, how I dreaded those monthly, then bi-weekly, then weekly check-ups because they included internal exams. I hate them, hate them, *hate* them. Always have, still do. They got increasingly more uncomfortable as my pregnancy progressed, but I thought it was a small price to pay to have a good birth. I would have some bleeding after each examination and thought on two occasions I thought the spotting meant I had lost the mucous plug. My last visit happened to be on my due date, and Dr. S seemed unusually concerned.

"Are you absolutely sure about your dates?" he asked.

"Yes. Why? Is there a problem?"

"Are your periods regular? How long is your cycle?"

"Isn't the due date just an estimate and any time two weeks before or after is still normal?"

"Yes, but we don't like you to go too long. There are more risks involved. We will consider an induction if you haven't had the baby by next week."

I couldn't understand what he was so worried about. I wasn't even over due yet.

Labour Day

It was three days past my due date and I had been up to the toilet for the third time during the night. I couldn't wait for the baby to be born. The constant pressure on my bladder was annoying and forced me out of bed to the bathroom every two hours. I was tired of it, tired of being pregnant, tired of being huge, and desperate for an uninterrupted night's sleep. (Stupid me, thinking that I'd get uninterrupted sleep *after* the baby was born!)

As I climbed back into bed I felt a "pop," like a thud, deep in my pelvis, followed by a trickle of warm water in my vagina.

"Bert! I think my water just broke!"

Bert startled, and leaped out of bed. As I reached over to turn on the light, hot water gushed out from me, flooding the bed. Oh, my! This is it! This is the big day! How exciting! How terrifying! What happens now? What should we do first? Isn't it wonderful we just put that plastic cover over the mattress today?

The doctor had said to come to the hospital when the contractions were five minutes apart or immediately if my water broke. We called my mother to let her know we were on our way. It was 3:30 a.m.

I shivered most of the way in the car partly from nervous excitement and partly because it was an icy February morning. I felt my first mild contractions on the way to the hospital.

We were happy to find we could get the birthing room, but what a disappointment to find out the "birthing room" was really just an operating room with wallpaper. Cold gray tiles covered the walls almost to the ceiling. The untiled part at the top of the walls was decorated with ugly yellow flowered wallpaper. A high, narrow bed dominated the centre of the room under an enormous round spotlight. Near the bed a yellow vinyl armchair blended with the ugly wallpaper. Opposite the window, which looked out onto a brick wall, was a glass and steel cabinet, which hid the birth instruments behind a plain green fabric. This was their attempt at a home-like atmosphere?

I was questioned and examined by a yawning resident who looked like he hadn't slept for days. I was grateful Dr. S had given permission to be up walking. Many doctors did not allow patients to be out of bed at all with ruptured membranes because of the risk of infection.

So there was nothing else to do but wait until the delivery.

And wait.

And wait.

I was allowed to walk around, but there was nowhere to go. I was allowed to go only as far as the waiting/smoking/TV room, where smokers, with nothing else to do, would stare at this wandering pregnant woman. Every time I went in the hall, the friendly chatter among the staff abruptly ceased, as they waited for me to walk past them. Then they'd resume their conversation in hushed voices. So I spent most of the time in my room, bored.

We chatted about how nice it would be to soon be bringing the new baby home. We agreed on names: Joshua if a boy, Victoria if a girl. I had brought a book to read and playing cards to occupy my time like I was going on some sort of a picnic, but we were pretty excited about the whole adventure, too excited to get involved in any games. Besides, there were too many interruptions for cards or reading.

The Childbirth Classes hadn't taught me to just keep busy and ignore the contractions as long as possible, they taught us we must concentrate on our breathing to keep on top of the contractions, "In Control" at all times lest the pains get ahead of us. I was doing my breathing correctly as I had been taught, even though the contractions were mild and could easily have been ignored.

Several medical students and nurses took turns examining me every hour or so. Each time, Bert would be asked to leave the room. I guess it was uncomfortable for the doctor to have the husband watch his wife spread her legs for a stranger with a probing gloved hand. I consented to all these exams because I decided to be a nice cooperative patient by letting them learn on me. Dr. S said he thought I'd have the baby about noon. How exciting!

After a lunch from the "clear fluids only" menu (Jell-O and apple juice), Dr. S announced I was six centimetres dilated. Over halfway to full dilation! My labour was getting stronger, and it was all back labour. I lay on the narrow bed and Bert rubbed my back until his arms ached. I tried knee-chest position, which helped a bit. However, lying on the chest with one's butt up in the air, particularly in a backless Patient Uniform leaves one in a rather embarrassing position. Staff members seem to be allowed to walk in unannounced at any time, and do, so while it was physically more comfortable, I could not relax in a position that embarrassed me. At 4:00 in the afternoon I was still at six centimetres. Though discouraged because labour was taking so long, I was still handling the contractions well.

Dr. S, however, wasn't handling it well. He was concerned about the lack of progress and gave me a deadline. If things weren't better by suppertime, he said, he would consult his colleague about my case.

I was so downhearted I felt like crying. What was wrong? Why was it taking so long? What were they going to do about "my case"?

I sat down in the cold yellow vinyl armchair and resolved to concentrate more on relaxation, letting go and allowing my body do its work, as taught in childbirth class. Relax I did; falling sound asleep in the armchair between contractions, my head drooping forward. The contraction would wake me and I would lean forward to unstick my body from the vinyl and rub my lower back during the pains. I napped this way for a couple of hours.

At suppertime I was given a delightful meal of a half-cup of Jell-O and black tea (I take mine with milk). A nurse checked me and said I was at eight centimetres. Great news! Then the resident took his turn between my legs, and turning to the nurse, sharply corrected her. "She's *six*." My heart sank. No progress at all. It was time to call in the troops about "my case." *What is wrong with me?* I wondered.

The Battle of all Mothers

Dr. N. was pulling on his rubber glove as he entered the room. Without making eye contact, he introduced himself to me at the same moment he introduced his fingers into my vagina. Then he explained the battle plan. For the first line of attack, I had to have an epidural. An epidural? I always thought the epidural was for women who couldn't handle the pain, but I was handling the pain fine. I was taught it should be avoided because it tends to slow labour down, but the doctor explained it could be an effective tool for natural childbirth: Many mothers are just too tense and uptight, he said, and by removing the pain, the epidural helps them relax. Once they relax, the body can do its work more effectively, so they dilate faster, and can soon have their baby, naturally. He told me with grave concern of his trouble with the time factor, since the risk of infection increases the longer the membranes have been ruptured.

Feeling defeated, I reluctantly accepted the epidural. There was no other option offered. The minute the doctor left the room I broke down and sobbed. I did not want the epidural. I wanted natural childbirth. I felt like I'd lost the battle before I even got to the front lines.

A nurse tried to comfort me, or help get me back In Control saying, "We don't give out medals here for being a martyr." I shouldn't feel like a failure, she said, after all, lots of women who were planning natural childbirth break down and end up taking the epidural. But I *didn't* break down! I didn't *want* it! The doctor wouldn't do this unless he had to, would he? He knew how important it was to me to have this baby naturally, didn't he? It must be for the best; it must be the only way. What could I do but trust him?

Two interns and a nurse sent Bert down to get supper while they put the epidural in my back. It hurt! I was positioned on my side facing the glass cabinet. In the glass door I could see the reflections of the two interns at my back. After feeling the needle being inserted what felt like several inches into my spine, I could see them standing there, their arms folded, looking at my back. *What on earth were they doing*, I wanted to know.

"We're waiting," was their reply. *Waiting? Waiting for what?* The back pain was worse than ever, each contraction causing me to move and wriggle and writhe from the pain. I wanted them to get the damn epidural working NOW! Once you have given up the fight, you can't get the epidural fast enough. There's no point in suffering any more.

"Stop moving around," they scolded me. I was in agony, trying to keep from moving during the contractions. They wouldn't explain what they were doing to me, and got very irritated by my questions. They snapped at me to hold still. Hold still? I'd like to see them try to hold still during a back labour, with a steel rod in the spine!

The effect of the epidural was like warmth going from my waist to my toes. The contractions reduced to a tight numbness, a buzzing sensation more than a cramp. It surprised me, because I had always heard women say they were "dead from the waist down." I could still move my legs.

With the epidural, of course, I had to have an IV. And the baby had to be watched closely by means of an internal fetal monitor. I gritted my teeth to keep from screaming as the doctor put his fist up inside me and screwed an electrode into my baby's scalp, grateful at the moment for the numbing effect of the epidural! A second tube inserted beside the baby's head measured the strength of the contractions. I wept softly throughout these procedures, biting my knuckle, trying my best to stay "in control."

Little did I know at the time, I had already lost control. It took my VBAC to realize, being in control is not about giving birth without moaning or yelling or crying out in pain; that's *normal*. Being in control is about being in charge of the environment, asserting oneself in the situation, and having a sense of personal power over decisions. I was in control, all right: in their control!

Just as I had read and learned in Childbirth Class, the epidural slowed down my labour. I later wondered: if the Childbirth Education Instructor knew the epidural slows labour down, surely the doctor did. Why would he order an epidural as a treatment for a slow labour?

Dr. N quickly moved in to the front line of the battleground, bringing out the heavy artillery to show my uterus just who was in command. He ordered a urinary catheter for me, making a total of three tubes and wires sticking out of what I had formerly considered "private parts." Then they brought in the "pump," a machine designed to push synthetic hormones into my veins to contract my uterus. Contract it did, so much it wouldn't let up its grip on my baby, and the monitor showed the baby was in distress. The nurse jumped up, dropping her chart to the floor, flipped me over onto my side, and slapped an oxygen mask on my face. She turned the pump down, and we all breathed a sigh of relief when the baby's heart rate returned to normal. But the contractions stopped. She turned up the pump again to stimulate more contractions, and again the baby went into distress.

I was totally disheartened. I wished I'd never had the epidural; it seemed to make everything worse. I had no options any more, but to do as they said. I felt like running away, but I was confined to bed, rails up to prevent me from falling out, wires and tubes connecting me to poles and bags and machines. Everyone was focused on the monitor, watching, listening to the beeps and blips. As each contraction would register on the monitor, we would hold our breath, watching as the contraction caused the baby's heart-rate to slow, dipping lower and lower on the computer readout, closer and closer to the danger zone. The contraction would end, and Bert, the nurse, and I would sigh with relief, listening to the beep-beep-beep of the baby's heartbeat, stable once again.

I was no longer a labouring woman; I was a dangerous environment holding a baby hostage. Everything was my fault: my body wouldn't do what it was supposed to, trapping the baby inside me. The doctors, the nurses, my family, everyone, was waiting for me. It was my fault everyone was so tired. I felt so bad, keeping the doctor up late, keeping my family waiting. I was so sorry I had done this to them. My mother and my sister had been sitting all day long in the waiting room; worrying, knitting to pass the time, and waiting for me to produce the first grandchild. Poor Bert was worn out, and stressed to the limit. When he was close to me I could tell sometime within the last 12 hours, driven by the stress of the situation, he had taken up the habit of smoking again.

It was 21 hours since my membranes had ruptured. Twenty-four hours and the risk of infection is increased substantially, the obstetrician had warned. There was only one thing left to do to get everyone out of this nightmare. The nurse handed me a clipboard and a pen to sign consent for the cesarean section. "Change the date," I sighed, handing the paper back, "It's after midnight."

The option of whether to be awake or asleep for the surgery was left up to me. I knew it was best to be awake but I was so frightened: I could still feel the contractions, and if this was what women called "dead from the waist down," I sure didn't want to be cut open and feel it!

"Whatever you want to do, Doctor," I answered, "Whatever you think is best." I knew exactly what he would choose, and hated myself for being so weak and frightened. I knew it would be easier for him and the staff if I was not conscious. For me, it meant sweet oblivion, an escape from this nightmare of worrying. There would be no more endless waiting, no more wondering about the baby. Someone else would take care of all the problems and I didn't have to face it anymore. If I surrendered, the war would soon be over.

As I was wheeled out of the birthing room I caught one last look at Bert before the doors swung shut. There stood my husband alone in the room where we had spent our last few hours as a childless couple, alone with only his fear for his wife and baby. I never saw him looking so anxious and defeated, unable to do anything but watch, helpless, as they wheeled me away. No one put an arm around his shoulder to tell him it would be all right.

Everyone was bustling about in the operating room, preparing for the surgery. The operating room staff chatted cheerfully amongst themselves as they went about their work, putting a mask over my face, shaving the top part of my pubic hair and coating my belly with antiseptic. I felt like a great enormous turkey being prepared for a banquet. I was terrified they might forget I wasn't asleep and would cut me open, so I continued to talk non-stop, an inaudible mumble through the mask.

It was hard to breathe flat on my back, the full weight of my uterus on top of me. My legs were immobilized, strapped to the operating table. A paper cap was placed over my hair. My arms were both outstretched on boards, one for a blood pressure cuff, one pierced with the IV. The doctor poised his hand over me, scalpel ready. *My God! Have they forgotten me?* Soon I'd be 'dead to the world' and they would pierce my belly, and blood and water would flow out. As a welcome oblivion flooded my mind, it occurred to me that I was being crucified.

Welcome to Motherhood

Through a dark fog of muffled voices, a woman was crying, sobbing like her heart was broken. Just a lonely voice, crying in the wilderness. Someone was trying to soothe her. *It's okay*, the soothing voice said, *we've given you something for the pain*. What pain? Who is talking? I don't understand the words in the swirling dark fog, and I can't see.

"Wake up, Sheila," the voice said again, "You have a baby boy." The heartbroken woman sobbed and I felt a sharp pain. Why am I hurting? The fog slowly began to slip away, clearing my mind, and I recognized the heartbroken sobs in the dark void; they were my own. And the pain was mine too, growing sharper as the fog cleared, overwhelming. I tried to stop the crying, for the jerking sobs sent stabbing pains through my belly.

I reached down to touch my tummy, covered with thick bandages. It was empty, soft, the life gone from inside me. *Where did you go, little one?*

"He has red hair!" It was Bert's voice, but his words didn't make sense to me. Who has red hair? The baby? We both have dark hair. They've made a mistake. Where would my husband and I get a baby with red hair?

Bert's voice sounded close to me, proud and happy. I couldn't see him through the fog. I wanted to see the smile I heard in my husband's voice but I couldn't see through the tears as they ran over my nose into my other eye and down my cheek to the pillow. I didn't know it, but while I was asleep the nurse had taken my thumbprint (and the baby's footprint) for the hospital birth certificate. In my still-drugged stupor I smeared black ink from my thumb raccoon-like across my face as I attempted to wipe away my tears.

On the way from Recovery to my room they stopped the stretcher at the nursery so I could see the baby. The babies' heads were all facing west; my head was facing east. I tried to sit up to make sense of the squirming pink backward upside-down wiggling blobs of flesh. With my vision still blurred, all I could see were aquariums containing what appeared to be piglets.

The delivery room nurses helped the maternity nurses get me into bed, and then bustled about adjusting the IV pole, the blood pressure cuff, the bedding and pillows. One of them washed the ink off my face and hands, then spread my legs, washed my genital area and put a sanitary napkin on me. I wished I were still unconscious.

I was still crying. The nurse wanted to know what was wrong, but the fog in my mind wouldn't let me form the words. She could only assume I needed more pain medication. But physical pain wasn't the reason for my tears. So far, becoming a mother had been very much like becoming a car accident victim several years earlier when both my legs were broken. Every inch of my body ached; every movement caused pain. The shock and the drugs and the confusion and the disappointment and the fear and the relief couldn't be expressed. I could only cry.

One nurse wisely decided I needed to hold my baby. She soon presented to me a tightly wrapped blue and white striped blanket, out of which appeared a red face.

"Can I nurse him?"

"You can try, but I don't think he'll be interested right now."

I desperately wanted to breastfeed this baby. I just *had* to. I had failed at childbirth and I needed to feel like I mattered to the baby, like I could do something special nobody else could do. It had taken an entire team of medical staff to get him out of me; I hoped I could at least feed him by myself. The nurse struggled to get me sitting upright then arranged pillows behind me and under my arms. Being careful of the IV and covering the incision with another pillow, we managed to wrestle a boob out of the backless Patient Uniform, and get the baby in my arms, an exercise that exhausted me. The sleepy baby ignored me completely. The nurse said not to worry; they had probably already fed him in the nursery. *Oh, great,* I thought, *someone even has to look after feeding it.*

Bert and my family had all gone home to bed. It was 24 hours since the nightmare had begun at home in my own bed. I wished Bert were with me. In my private room, I realized I was totally alone for the first time in months. How desperately I missed the life inside my belly! How I longed for the slow, stretching movements, the sharp kicks, and the rhythmic tap-tap-tap inside my belly I recognized as hiccups. My belly was empty, my arms were empty, my heart empty too. *I'll feel better if I get some sleep*, I thought.

I was still crying when the sun came up.

* * *

Things were better in the morning. The nurse brought the baby and stood over me, watching to make sure I would get him latched on properly. I asked if it would be all right to leave me alone with the baby. I simply wanted privacy to fumble through this nursing thing by myself. I assured her I would call her if I needed help. Luckily, the baby took to breastfeeding like an old pro. He was brought to me every four hours for feedings two minutes on each breast, and then back to the nursery[i]. I held the baby and marveled at the miracle of this new life: a new being; part of me, part of my husband, symbolizing our one-ness, what God hath joined together.

During one of these feeding times the obstetrician came to see me accompanied by a team of medical students. With the baby in my arms and my heart bursting with awe and emotion for this sweet new life, I thanked Dr. N for doing the surgery and for giving me my beautiful healthy baby.

Much later I realized what a profound impact my little speech must have had on the medical students. They would have seen Dr. N as a hero! Like a knight in shining armor, he had rescued this damsel

---

[i] Four-hour feeding schedules are a hospital invention having little to do with what babies and mothers need, and much to do with running an institution on schedule. Keep your baby with you and feed him ridiculously often. Two-minute limits do *not* prevent nipple soreness as was thought, but do prevent proper stimulation of hormones to activate a plentiful milk supply.

in distress and saved the innocent child from the brink of death. We were going to live happily ever after, all thanks to him. And I, the fair maiden, was smiling and thanking him for cutting me open with his mighty sword, and rescuing my baby from the fierce dragon! Who wouldn't want to become an obstetrician, and be knighted with such power and glory?

The third day after surgery I was finally allowed food. The IV was removed and I could go have a shower. I locked the door and had a good look in the full-length mirror at my bruised, naked body. What a sight! A puffy red incision line, like a thin red mouth, smirked[i] at me over a goatee of partly-shaved pubic hair! Over a belly-button nose, two hugely swollen breasts protruded like mocking cartoon eyes!

My face was very pale, but a purplish bruise surrounded my eyes. The nurses suggested it might be a reaction to the drugs, but it looked like I'd been beaten up.

My mother came to visit when I was feeding the baby, and to my surprise, she did something I had not done yet: she unwrapped him and put him in my arms! Wow! How different it felt to hold and nurse a real baby! With arms and legs! Until then it was simply too awkward and uncomfortable for me. Simply getting my sore body into position to feed the baby was painful and exhausting. Every four hours I had dutifully fed the little red face in the tightly-wrapped blue-striped blanket, and handed the bundle back to the nurse. I was also scared to unwrap it, because they had warned me the baby was to be kept warm. I was afraid I'd get too exhausted part way through the task, wrap it incorrectly and Something Terrible would happen!

That evening, while holding the real-baby-with-arms-and-legs in my lap, I felt a familiar rhythmic tap-tap-tap against my belly. Hiccups! My baby! I looked down in amazement and sudden recognition: *It's YOU!* And for the first time, I knew in my heart this was MY baby! It was our little long-awaited baby Joshua, and finally he was here.

Cesarean Recovery

Recovering from both childbirth and major surgery is a physical challenge and an emotional roller coaster. Whenever I mentioned to anyone how sad I was about having a cesarean, I would get a stern lecture on how lucky I was to be living in an era when women didn't

---

[i] The scar was uneven, turned slightly up on the side where the obstetrician had stood while cutting; hence the smirk.

die in childbirth. I dared not bring it up again, so I put emotional recovery out of my mind in order to deal with my physical recovery.

Like any surgical patient, it was difficult to move from a lying to sitting position, or from a chair to standing, which I had to do often in order to feed the baby. I was not allowed to get in a bath until the scar healed or to lift "anything heavier than the baby." The lochia, or post-partum bleeding, lasted over six weeks. The scar across my belly was sore for several weeks, making it painful to laugh, cough, or sneeze.

Recovering from surgery is tiring. Looking after a newborn who nurses every two hours around the clock is relentless. Doing both at the same time is debilitating.

As much as I deeply loved the baby and took good care of him, I was exhausted, and even resentful of the demands on me from the baby, and then felt guilty for feeling resentment. How unfair for the poor baby. Days and nights all ran together in an endless longing for uninterrupted sleep. One night we tried saving my milk in a bottle so Bert could feed him and I could stay in bed. After one night we decided it wasn't worth the hassle: it took almost an hour to get a few ounces of milk into a bottle, and then when the baby roused I had to thump Bert (several times!) to wake him up. I lay there and listened to Bert trying to keep the baby relatively quiet while the bottle warmed up. *This is ridiculous*, I thought, *I could have fed the baby and come back to bed by now*. We decided from then on I would be responsible for night shift, but Bert would have to take up more of the daytime responsibilities.

I was thankful Bert was home and could take turns walking a fussy baby. We even pulled the couch away from the wall so we had room to pace the floor in circles. I couldn't imagine how I would have managed without him to take over when I was exhausted and in tears, feeling like a hopeless failure as a mother for being unable to stop my baby's crying. With horror I began to comprehend for the first time how some women, driven beyond the limits of endurance through sleep deprivation, emotional depression and physical exhaustion, could abuse their babies.

At the six weeks check-up the doctor said to my great relief the baby was doing just fine. I was so happy. At least, if I couldn't birth, I could breastfeed well! Bert was pretty happy too, because to *his* great relief the doctor also gave us permission to resume intercourse. He had a big dumb grin on his face and was ready to park the car on the way home from the doctor's and jump into the back seat with me. I'd sooner have jumped out the window.

Second Base

Getting a "feel" for it

CHAPTER 4

Everything I Needed to Know about Birthing, I Learned from Breastfeeding

> For you will nurse and be satisfied at her comforting breasts; you will drink deeply and delight in her overflowing abundance.
>
> \- Isaiah 66:11

Leche is a Spanish word, pronounced *lay-chay.* In English it means "milk." I learned this from watching *Sesame Street.*

La Leche League was the name chosen by the world's foremost organization on breastfeeding, because when it had its humble beginnings in 1956, people didn't use the word "breast" in polite company. The name was actually taken from a shrine built in honour of "Our Lady of Happy Delivery and Plentiful Milk."

La Leche League, the rumours said, was a bunch of fanatics who made you breastfeed until kindergarten. Since a local chapter of La Leche League met in my town, I wanted to go out of curiosity. I hoped nobody would put a gun to my head and force me to breastfeed longer than I had planned.

Putting my two-month old baby in a stroller, I walked the few blocks to the meeting, which was held on a weekday morning in someone's home. Tricycles and wagons and riding toys greeted me on the porch, and a big sign was taped to the door, "La Leche League — Please walk in."

There were four or five other women in the house, some with babies on their hips, chatting and looking over a library of books spread out on the kitchen table. Books! New books I hadn't seen at the local library! Books on parenting, books on discipline, books on childbirth and nutrition and on subjects I had never heard of, like The Family Bed by Tine Thevenin.

We sat down in the living room amidst toys and baby paraphernalia, babies on our laps. Someone passed around a tray of juice and the meeting began with a short description of the history of La Leche League.

I learned how the organization was started in 1956 by a group of young mothers like us, in a living room like this, where mothers met with their friends to offer information, encouragement and support for breastfeeding. I was assured La Leche League was not in the business of trying to "sell" breastfeeding. It was only there for the mother who *wanted* to breastfeed. Nobody was going to put a gun to my head after all.

The discussion topic was Advantages of Breastfeeding. We were asked to introduce ourselves and mention one way we had found breastfeeding to be particularly helpful. I thought about how nice it was to know that even if I couldn't give birth without surgery, at least I was giving my baby my own milk. Breastfeeding made me feel important to the baby, because it was something that only I could do. I guessed that this was what "bonding" meant; feeling like I really mattered to the baby.

When my turn came to talk, I introduced myself and said breastfeeding had helped me bond to the baby, because I'd been unconscious when he was born by cesarean section — and then my voice suddenly cracked and I burst into tears. I felt like such a fool. Here I was, crying in front of a bunch of strangers about a cesarean which had occurred two months ago! I was terribly embarrassed by my lack of self-control. Everyone in the room exchanged awkward glances in an uncomfortable silence. I wiped my nose on my sleeve. *I'm not over this yet!* I realized.

Not one person lectured me or implied I was not grateful for my healthy baby. They simply understood my pain, as well as my delight in my baby.

I enjoyed meeting and chatting with other moms about my breastfeeding concerns, and was relieved to discover other babies also want to nurse almost non-stop in the evenings, and other moms also face discouraging comments from friends and family. In spite of the common "Breast is best" adage, we still live in a culture where bottle-feeding is the norm. Most of the recent studies done on babies, like sleep patterns and weight gain, were done on bottle-fed babies. Many people worry, for instance, when the breastfed baby doesn't have bowel movements like the bottle-fed counterpart. I was surprised to learn the normal breastfed baby may only poop once a week.

While we talked, I noticed the most adorable little boy with big brown eyes and lashes anyone would covet. His mother had just finished nursing a baby about the same age as mine. The little boy toddled over to his mom, climbed on her lap without letting go of his toy, and flopped himself down into a nursing position. She lifted the bottom of her blouse, reached inside a moment to unhook her bra, and the little boy's dark curls shifted as he latched on to her breast. I couldn't believe it. Nursing *two*?

Crazy people, I thought, *Nice, but definitely fanatical.* One La Leche League meeting was enough to convince me the LLL members were a little crazy. It made no sense to me. Why keep breastfeeding a child who could walk and was learning to talk? Couldn't the baby take a cup by then? Why would they keep them babies for so long? It couldn't be good for them.

However, a month later, I found myself meeting in the same living room with the crazy breastfeeding fanatics. I went back because I was encouraged and intrigued by their cheerful attitude and obvious joy they had in mothering. I went back because they were willing to listen to an exhausted new mother complain about fatigue without blaming all her problems on nursing. I went back because they said I was doing a wonderful job of mothering by responding to my own baby as an individual. Good mothering, they pointed out, is about responding to the baby, not the clock. Besides, I had to go back: I had taken out almost half of the books they had available in their small library.

In spite of their extreme viewpoint on long-term nursing, there was something different about their attitude towards their babies, something that was delightfully refreshing. These women just seemed to *enjoy* their babies so much! Most people I spoke with considered breastfeeding to be a physically and emotionally draining obligation, something bravely endured because it was noble. One might cheerfully tolerate the inconvenience of breastfeeding a few months because it was the right thing to do, like going to the dentist, not something you did because it was enjoyable. La Leche League women actually seemed to downright *like* it, and they admitted it! They talked about breastfeeding as a wonderful, fulfilling expression of our femininity, an enchanting time to be savoured and enjoyed before it is gone forever.

I was curious. How does one learn to enjoy having to stop everything and feed a screaming child every two hours around the clock, for *months*? Can you actually appreciate being tied down so much? Can you learn to like leaking breasts? Wearing lumpy breast pads? Sore nipples?

I continued to attend La Leche League meetings for the next few months, to borrow all their books and learn all their secrets, but certainly not to be considered one of *them*, one of the fanatics. Not me. I planned on nursing my baby for one year, period. You wouldn't catch me breastfeeding a child who could walk and was learning to talk.

It was interesting to find out a bit about La Leche League's history. When it began, bottle-feeding was the standard way most babies were fed. "Yuck, why would you want to do *that*?" was the attitude. Modern, sophisticated women didn't do *that*, only animals or people who were too poor to afford the new, more civilized and superior method of feeding.

The new improved method of feeding even had a nice scientific name — Formula — because it was based on scientific calculations of nutritional requirements. Mothers were proud to feed their babies the modern way, showing their love and devotion to their babies through meticulous adherence to doctor's orders, carefully sterilizing the bottles and nipples, and feeding according to the strict schedule the doctor had recommended.

But some women did still want to breastfeed. They also followed their doctors' instructions carefully, adhering to a strict regime, washing their hands and nipples carefully before each scheduled breast-feeding. But if they had problems with their method of feeding, they had to quit. Nobody knew how to solve breastfeeding problems, and therefore it was assumed women had "evolved" to the point they were "too nervous" to feed their offspring like the lower animals. After an entire generation of women had enjoyed the freedom from the obligation of breastfeeding, the womanly art of breastfeeding had all but dried up.

Those who did breastfeed generally kept quiet about it because of the prevailing attitude. Breastfeeding was animalistic, or represented a poor standard of living, being unable buy the best for their babies. Things began to change at a church picnic in 1956 when Mary White and Marian Thompson were quietly sitting under a tree nursing their babies. They were chatting as women do about birth and babies and breastfeeding, and were surprised by women who would approach them with admiration, commenting wistfully how they wished they had been able to breastfeed too. So many mothers they knew had tried to breastfeed but only found frustration and failure, simply because they had no one to turn to for information and support. Helping mothers, they decided, would help families, and helping families would ultimately help the community. They decided there had to be a way to help.

They called up some of their friends who had also breastfed their babies, and with enthusiastic support from two local doctors they decided to hold a mothers meeting to share with their pregnant friends the secrets of successful breastfeeding. Since some of them had met with disaster in their previous attempts at breastfeeding, they knew the ability to breastfeed easily was not just a matter of getting "lucky."

This simple mother-to-mother sharing turned out to be exactly what the mothers needed to be able to successfully nurse their babies. The meetings grew and grew as more and more women found out about them. They didn't set out to become the world's most recognized authority on breastfeeding; all they ever expected was a get-together to help a few friends.

But while hordes of women were learning how to happily nurse their babies, right from the start this itty-bitty titty committee was considered radical. Not only because they were nursing their babies like animals do, instead of using the superior formulas, but because they suggested some outrageous ideas. For example, they told mothers they didn't need *any* bottles if they were breastfeeding! Unheard of! Surely the baby would starve! Not even *water*? What about juice for vitamin C requirements? Furthermore, these crazy mothers would give their babies nothing but breast milk, for *six months,* at a time when most babies were getting solid foods by six weeks!

In spite of the current medical practice of separating mothers from their newborns for up to twenty-four hours after birth, the kooky La Leche League women insisted mothers and babies *needed* each other right after birth. And to top things off, they even said it was better if women were *awake* during childbirth. Imagine! What kind of a weirdo would want to go through *that* if she didn't have to?

Yet all these kooky ideas are now commonly accepted norms. The changes you see today were brought about, not by doctors, but by people like you and me asking for what was rightly ours in the first place. Mothers and fathers who only wanted the best for their babies challenged their doctors. When doctors were forced to provide evidence their practices were helpful, their own studies confirmed the women's instincts had been right after all. Surprise! The milk in your breasts is superior to the formula the scientist made. Surprise! Your baby doesn't need any more vitamin C than what is already in your milk. Surprise! Mothers bond better with their babies when they are allowed to see them! After science proves women's instincts are correct, they then publish the information as though it was their idea first!

Even today, even with all the information available in print, on TV and the Internet, the ideal way for a mother to learn to happily breastfeed is the way it has been done for generations: by sharing information, encouragement, and support, mother to mother. La Leche League does not place their main focus on Hospital Seminars or TV advertisements. Meeting with another mother over a cup of tea and a muffin is the way we women operate: sharing, talking, and learning by example.

I know I learned a lot by example. I was amazed at my first LLL meeting as I watched the hostess, a mother of three small children, strap the baby into a front carrier and go into the kitchen to make egg-salad sandwiches. It had never occurred to me to use my carrier at home! I always thought those carriers were for use at the mall or when walking somewhere a stroller wouldn't go. I had spent most of my daily waking hours trying to get things done while the baby slept. It was frustrating because I couldn't simply ignore his cries, and I couldn't hold him and get my work done.

From then on, my carrier got endless hours of use. My baby was happier. Snug in his carrier and contented by my presence, he didn't fuss as much. I was happier. I had hands free to get my housework done. Rather than feeling burdened, I began to enjoy the cuddly feeling of having the baby close, involved in my everyday activities, watching everything contentedly from his little papoose. Surprisingly, I didn't feel like the baby interrupted my life as much, even though he was with me more. Admittedly, it got tiring at times, but it was a welcome trade-off for the frustration both the baby and I had felt before. Some call the baby carrier a "womb with a view."

Another thing I noticed about La Leche League women was how frequently they nursed their babies. They often nursed even more than I did, and I had thought every two hours was excessive. Rather than trying to figure out what the baby was fussing about, they just offered the breast, and often the babies would nurse for a minute or two and be happy again. It didn't make sense: everyone else I knew worked at scheduling the baby into nursing *less*. These women nursed *more*, and yet didn't seem to mind a bit.

When my baby was about six months old, a new mom came to the La Leche League meeting with lots of questions and concerns and worries. As I chatted with her I realized I was now the more experienced mother, the one supporting her through those exhausting early weeks. It felt good to be able to offer her the same encouragement that had been given to me. By now I understood the secrets to successful breastfeeding.

I no longer worried about how often my baby nursed, and had long since quit thinking of nursing as "feeding," realizing it is so much more than just a source of nutrition. Breast milk comes as a package wrapped in mommy's soft arms and familiar voice, her own special smell, and her loving eyes gazing into the baby's. The whole package is love; milk is merely a bonus product of the relationship. When we see nursing as a love relationship, not just a feeding method, we see recognized love flows best when given freely. We would not keep track of how often or how long we nurse the baby any more than we would keep track of how often we kiss and cuddle the baby.

Loving the baby freely and fully in this manner deepens the bond between mother and child, and ultimately affects the decision of how to go about weaning the baby. The day he turned one he learned to walk, and my baby did not appear any less adorable, any less in need of the loving comfort and warm cuddliness of nursing, than he had the day before his birthday. And on his first birthday, wrapped in kisses and snuggling, curled up in my arms he was nursed to sleep as usual, oblivious to the culture which would frown so disapprovingly at his suckling — and labeling his mother officially as a crazy fanatical mother of a nursing toddler who could walk and was learning to talk.

Breastfeeding the Easy Way, Learning the Hard Way

Any new mother is unsure of herself, but most of us wouldn't dare admit it and appear inept. Each of us wants to be the best mother in the world. With the first baby everything is new, everything you do is an adjustment.

We live in a culture in which baby bottles are a much more common representation of baby care than lactating breasts. Having grown up in a generation where breast-feeding is not the norm, many new mothers get little support from their own families for their decision to do so, especially if the grandparents did not breastfeed. Family and friends mean well, but they may not know how to offer support, and may not understand how vulnerable the new mother is to discouraging comments. Negative comments, however subtle, can make one feel burdened by breastfeeding. Innocent comments and questions can cause the oversensitive new mother to doubt herself, or her decision to breastfeed:

"You must be awfully tied down." *I can't go anywhere without the baby. I have to lug him around all the time.*

"Does he sleep through the night yet? Mine slept through at three weeks." *He'd sleep better if I gave him formula.*

"You must be exhausted, nursing so often" *I'm tired, and it's because I'm breastfeeding.* (Really, it's hardly exhausting to sit down and put your feet up and watch TV while the baby nurses.)

"It's too bad your husband can't feed him." *I'm depriving my husband and the baby of a close relationship.*

"Are you allowed to eat that / drink that / do that when you are nursing?" *Will I ruin my milk? Will I hurt my baby?*

"Why is he crying? You must have eaten something that doesn't agree with him." *It's my fault the baby is fussy.*

"You're feeding him again? Didn't you just feed him a while ago?" *There's something wrong with a baby who has to eat this often.*

"How do you know if he's getting enough?" *I don't know if he is getting enough.*

"Don't you ever give him a bottle so you can get away?" *I need to get away!*

"What would happen if you got sick?" *Oh my goodness the baby would starve if anything happened to me!*

"How long are you going to nurse?" *I'm still new at this, but I better start making plans for weaning.*

Before too long, the nursing mother has developed a "poor me" attitude. She considers everything she does in relation to breastfeeding. *Can I do that if I'm breastfeeding? Can I eat this? Drink that? Will it affect the baby? Will my milk dry up? What if I overfeed? Underfeed? What if I get sick? When will my life ever be the same?* She feels "different." She wants to get back to normal. She lives as if breastfeeding is an abnormality.

Interestingly, until the common use of birth control, and especially since the widespread use of the Pill, most women gave birth to and nursed several babies. Around the turn of the century the average Canadian woman had seven children. Breastfeeding and pregnancy were the normal state for married women until menopause. *Not* breastfeeding is really the abnormality.

The question we should be asking ourselves is not whether or not this or that is okay while one is breastfeeding, because lactation is what's supposed to happen after childbirth. We ought to be asking whether it is normal and healthy for women <u>not</u> to be pregnant and lactating throughout their childbearing years. What damage can result when we suppress lactation and conception and continue to menstruate every month for 30 to 40 years?

Simple Secrets of Successful Suckling

The following four points are the major misunderstood obstacles getting in the nursing mother's way. All of them interfere with the natural state of breastfeeding by adding unnecessary restrictions.

Raise four fingers of your right hand in a Suckling Salute, place your left hand over your breast, and repeat after me:

No Soothers
No Supplements
No Schedules
No Solids

These four simple secrets summarize steps to successful suckling. These simple standards stop snarls before they start, see.

1. No Soothers. (Pacifier or "dummy")

A mother of a four-month-old said she felt as if she didn't have enough milk any more, and wondered what she could do to stop herself from drying up. I told her, among other things, she should avoid using the soother. She had spent four months, she said rather unhappily, trying to get the baby to finally take one! I pointed out how her milk supply was ample until the baby started spending several hours a day sucking on the soother instead of her breast.

The soother is a great invention for bottle-fed babies who can't spend the day drinking from a bottle because they would get overfed. You can't over-feed a breastfed baby. A baby can regulate the amount of milk he takes from the breast by the way he sucks. Soothers are handy for use in the car or some other place where you just can't nurse and the baby just can't wait.

The breast makes as much milk as the baby tells it to make by his sucking. More sucking means more milk; less sucking, less milk. Therefore you can feed twins or triplets, because there is twice or thrice the amount of sucking being done at the breast. Reduce the sucking by overuse of the soother, and you give your body the signal it doesn't need to make as much milk.

The soother also introduces the risk of being used as a substitute, not just for mother's breast, but for mother. Substitutes harm the relationship. Babies need to be held. Mother needs to hold her baby, too. The close physical contact required by nursing affects the hormone levels which influence nurturing behaviour, as will be explained later.

2. No Supplements

For the same reason as stated above, you need to avoid supplementary bottles. If you give your baby a bottle instead of feed him, your body doesn't get the message to make milk. Mothers accidentally wean the baby this way. The occasionally bottle becomes a necessity when the breast isn't given the milk-making message. It's not nice to try to fool Mother Nature.

This is one of the big mistakes hospitals still make in sending home those free gift packs containing samples of formula. Along with the gift comes the implication you will probably need it. Any time you doubt your ability; the sample is ready to help when you doubt your own supply… which is exactly what the formula company wants! The only reason you are being given this "gift," is not because they love you dearly and want to make your life easier, but because they want you to doubt yourself and buy their product.

What mother doesn't have a bad day occasionally? She seems to have a million things to do, and the baby has fussed all day in spite of how often she feeds him; she is exhausted and suddenly she remembers the ready-to-serve gift sample of formula. She gives him a bottle, and sure enough, the baby sleeps for hours, proving — or so it appears — she doesn't have enough milk. Next day, the same thing happens. Even though she nurses him a lot, he still fusses, then remembering how well it worked before, she gives formula again. She doesn't intend to wean, but weaning is exactly what she is doing.

Perhaps she didn't have enough milk. But she needn't worry about it, because it's perfectly *normal*, and the remedy is not to quit nursing but to keep nursing, because increased nursing means increased production. Besides, the breast is never totally empty. The baby is frustrated because the *flow* of milk has decreased, but there is always another drop of milk. It's something like the way you can always squeeze another drop of urine from the bladder, even if you just "went," because the kidneys constantly produce urine. The breast is not like the bladder, though. The bladder is only a warehouse, while the breast is also a manufacturing site.

Lots of babies will nurse almost non-stop in the evenings in the early weeks. Hang in there. Take the phone off the hook and keep nursing and rocking and trying everything to get through the fussing. Don't expect to get anything done, you'll only get frustrated. And yes, it's frustrating! So grow up, already! Who said parenting would be easy? Talk to a friend who understands, but be selective about who you complain to, because many will still tell you the way to solve your breastfeeding problems is by bottle-feeding… which is like telling you to solve sexual problems by abstinence.

Try a nice brisk walk with the baby in a carrier. Try a car ride. Take a bath, with the baby. Though it's hard to believe at the time, try to remember: babies grow up very quickly. Why, before you know it, the fussing in the evenings will be replaced by arguing over bedtimes.

3. No Schedules

My friend Terry says she can't imagine Mary, the mother of Jesus, running outside to check the sundial every time Jesus wanted to nurse. Adults – who can understand the concept of delayed gratification, yet seldom go more than a couple of hours without a drink of water, coffee break, or snack – should not expect little babies to nurse only according to a clock they are too young to read.

Babies have periods of rapid growth, and may suddenly need extra nursing, the way an athlete needs extra fluids during a workout. Growth doesn't always occur in a regular manner, but in spurts, which is why strict schedules can be detrimental. Trust the baby when he seems to be extra hungry. When you are pregnant, you have days when you are ravenous for no apparent reason, too, but you know your body needs food to grow the baby. Even a teenage boy may be suddenly hungry all the time, though his body appears to be doing nothing more strenuous than playing video games.

The schedule is a man's invention imposed upon women.[i] Women are intuitive creatures, while men tend to have to see things in black and white. Women feed the baby when the baby seems to want it, or when she wants it - when her breasts feel like they need emptying.

Some people believe it is a good idea to get the baby onto a schedule because it will help the mother be better organized, and be able to accomplish more with her life without being at the beck and call of a demanding infant. You will either have to ignore his crying or will have to bounce him and rock him and give him a soother, distracting him any way you can to make him wait until it's "time" to nurse. Wouldn't it be easier just lifting your blouse and nursing for a few minutes?

The important thing is to look at *the baby*, not at the clock, to know when to nurse. By taking the focus off the baby and onto the clock, the schedule causes a rift between the mother and her baby. He's frustrated because he wants to nurse and she won't let him; she's frustrated because he's fussing and it's not feeding time. Nursing is a way to show love to your baby, because it makes him feel good inside and out. He adores you, for you are the world to him, being all he needs: the source of comfort and security and food and love. Don't let the clock hurt your relationship with your baby.

---

[i] Beware of books proclaiming unique "Baby wisdom." Be especially wary of any man who claims his method is "God's Way." The Bible says women are to learn about childcare from *women*! Titus2:3 (Remember the lifeguard who couldn't swim?)

4. No Solids.

There used to be a big push to get babies to eat solids early, for several reasons. Firstly, because babies need the added nutrition earlier if they weren't breastfed, and most weren't. Secondly, some believed the baby will sleep through the night if you stuffed it before bedtime. Thirdly, because people thought breastmilk alone was not sufficient. Finally, because babies would gag and sputter, it was presumed babies had to be taught how to eat, and the sooner the better. Those of us who wait until our babies are ready have found this to be untrue. My son had no solid food until he was seven months old and 23 pounds, when he leaned over in my lap and took a bite out of my cheese sandwich. He looked bewildered, ate it, and reached for more.

Those crazy La Leche League women who were telling women back in the 50's to wait about six months before they started solid foods, and pediatricians now recommend introduction of solids between four and six months of age. However, when mothers were surveyed over 20% of had started feeding solids *before* four months, and almost 70% were eating solids before six months of age.[14]

What most mothers do is ask their doctor when to start the baby on solid food. The doctor is simply basing his recommendations on what the Pediatric Society recommends, rather than on *your baby*. The four-to-six month range actually means bottle-fed babies should start solids around four months, and breastfed babies around six because their nutrition is superior.

Many mothers start the day the baby turns four months old. One worried lady asked me whether four months meant the same calendar date as his birth or the same weekday sixteen weeks after his birth. See the needless worry here? Feed your baby solids when *your baby* is ready. Put your eyes on the baby, not on the calendar!

The hard part, especially for the first time mother, is waiting, especially when all your peers have their babies on solid food, and your baby still is happy as a lark on nothing but your milk. If your four-month-old baby throws a fit when everyone is eating, try giving him a spoon and see if it was really just the spoon he wanted, not food. Because you are his mother, you know your baby better than the doctor does, or your neighbour, or your La Leche League Leader, or anyone else. You will become the expert on your child and see when he is ready for solid food. You see he is able to sit up by himself and put things into his mouth and bite and chew. He drools and can turn his head away when he's had enough. He uses his lips and/or tongue to make sounds. He suddenly increases his demand to be fed. It happens *sometime around* six months, and your baby will be different than every other baby.

5. No Sex

No, just kidding. It is very common though for women to find sex isn't very good for quite a while after the birth. And when you do attempt it, babies have an amazing radar system which immediately recognizes the moment mom's focus and hormones are slipping out of baby's range and into something a little more comfortable...

Experts Advise

Many women make the mistake of asking a doctor for advice on breastfeeding, though the doctor may not know much about it other than "Breast is best." Unless your doctor has breastfed, he may not know much about how to deal with the normal day-to-day common concerns and minor difficulties mothers face, most which are easily overcome. Breastfeeding problems are rarely due to medical problems. You don't need to ask a medical doctor a non-medical question.

Find out what your doctor knows about breastfeeding. Did his wife breastfeed? How long? How long does he think babies ought to be nursed? Does he agree with the World Health Organization's recommendation of breastfeeding for two years or more?

One doctor told me a lot of women – at *least* 10% according to him – aren't able to breastfeed. To say one in ten have lactation failure is like saying a one in ten people have kidney failure. Certainly there are abnormalities, but they are rare, far from the norm. Breastfeeding is a normal function.

Being a breastfeeding advocate, I asked the doctor how he knew for sure when women didn't have enough milk. He gave me an example. Last week, he said, a mother came in with her new baby. She was unsure of herself and didn't know if her baby is getting enough to eat. She's feeding every four hours like he told her to, to give her breasts time to "fill up" between feedings. *Wrong, wrong, wrong.*

In the office, the baby's weight gain was questionable, not surprisingly. The baby was not getting enough time at the breast to stimulate milk production! He told the mother to feed the baby, right then and there, to see how much milk she had. When the time was up, they weighed the baby again and *see*? Barely two ounces!

No wonder! What nervous new mother could perform under those circumstances? I'll bet if he stood over patients and made them pee a certain amount within a certain length of time he'd see a large percentage of kidney failure, too! She'd probably have been fine if he told her what a lovely, healthy baby she had, and what a great job she was doing, and to nurse her baby freely so she'd have lots of milk.

And no, he said, his wife had not breastfed any of their four children; she'd had no milk. Why?

Unfortunately, doctors are often the ones who tell a mother to quit breastfeeding, and many women would never question their doctors. If a woman is tearfully complaining about her breastfeeding concerns, the doctor might tell her to wean because he assumes that is what the mother *wants* to hear. He can instantly stop her worries about feeding by offering an alternative. Problem solved. Or it might be that he simply has no idea how to help her. He is not likely to have any experience with sore nipples or engorgement, a poor latch, or how to increase the milk supply. His job is to ensure the baby gained the right amount of weight, and he knows formula will get immediate results. He might tell her to wean if she has mastitis or the flu, because he has no idea of how to manage these problems. Women are usually told to wean if they have to take any medication, though it's usually not necessary. Many still make the mistake of advising the mother to offer a bottle after breastfeeding, to confirm the baby was satisfied at the breast.

Even though it violates the WHO code, many doctors still give out free formula samples to breastfeeding mothers, not realizing how it undermines their confidence in their ability. Some pediatricians advise feeding the baby only at scheduled intervals as a means of early discipline. They believe a baby should not be allowed to nurse whenever he wants or it will spoil him.

Parenting "experts" often advise you to never, ever allow the baby to nurse to sleep, as this supposedly prevents sleep problems later. This statement brings out the feminist in me. How dare some man — who has never experienced the joy of breastfeeding — deny a woman one of the most sensuously fulfilling moments she may ever experience as a mother? There is nothing as sweet as nursing a baby to sleep. I hope the expert's wife only allows him sex on a weekly schedule so he knows he can't expect it whenever he asks.

Formula for Disaster

Every formula claims to be the most like mother's milk. Even with the changes and improvements and new discoveries necessitating new additives, the baby-milk manufacturers have been making the same claim for over a hundred years!

Formula is a man's creation: a carefully calculated complex concoction of adequate nutrients for infants. It is given in measured amounts at measured times according to the weight of the infant. Babies were fed on schedules in hospitals because it was easier for the staff. Even in the 1800's some child-rearing experts recommended meals occur at regular intervals, so adults and infants alike were given the same rules. But breast milk is not like eating a steak. Its design assures quick, easy digestion in the human system and absorbed so well there is very little waste (which is the reason a breastfed baby can go several days without a bowel movement). Formula does keep babies feeling full longer, but longer satiation doesn't mean healthier. You would feel full longer after eating a pound of Oreo cookies than eating a pound of fruit, too, but which is healthiest?

Cow's milk is absolutely perfect by itself if your baby is a calf, weighs 150 pounds at birth and will be walking within a few minutes. Human milk is absolutely perfect for humans who need its species-specific enzymes for brain growth. Cow's milk is not used for formula because it's similar to human milk; it's used because of its cheap availability. Pig's milk is closer chemically to human milk.[15]

Not only is an artificial, man-made formula inferior to the custom-made milk the mother provides from her own body for her own baby, the act of bottle-feeding itself, *even if the baby receives breastmilk* in the bottle, is inferior to breastfeeding.

The mother controls bottle-feeding. She decides how much to feed the baby, and how often — or asks her doctor, who has even less contact with the child. Breastfeeding is a profoundly intimate relationship, the first intimate relationship a child has with another human being on this earth. In this reciprocal relationship the baby lets his mother know when he is hungry and signals her. She offers her breast, he takes it. He knows when he has had enough, and she doesn't coax him to take more as she may with a bottle. Nursing is a relationship based on communication between mother and child, while bottle-feeding is method of feeding based on measurements and calculations.

One woman asked me if it was not monotonous for the baby to have nothing but breastmilk for several months. She didn't understand there is a difference for the breastfed baby. While his bottle-fed counterpart tastes the same factory-made recipe day after day, the lucky breastfed baby's meal changes. The flavour changes according to what the mother eats, the amount increases according to the baby's needs, and the composition changes according to the seasons; having a higher water content in the hot summer months, and a higher fat content in the cold winter months. It even changes during the feeding, quenching the baby's thirst with the watery foremilk, gradually changing to a thicker, creamier dessert of hindmilk toward the end of the feeding.

You would think a substitute for the human breast might be a designed more like a breast: rounded in shape, perhaps something like a Hershey's Kiss. Catherine Young, in an editorial in Compleat Mother Magazine noted how the baby bottle, designed by men, is phallic in shape. Perhaps there was some subconscious satisfaction in the design, especially when seeing the child suck on it.

Another gender-bender of disturbing note was an advertisement for the "Baby Bonder" in Parenting Magazine in March 1988. This was nothing more than a terrycloth and fleece bib "designed to simulate the intimacy of infant nursing."

> *Simply insert a plastic bottle in either of the openings provided; fasten the bib around your neck; and it's feeding time... for one baby or two! Now fathers, working mothers, grandparents and close relatives can enjoy the all-important process of infant bonding. With Dr. Goldson's baby Bonder®, the only thing missing is a warm body, soft eye contact, and a familiar voice.*

"Now, nursing can be done by anyone for just $19.95," the ad stated. He claimed his baby had an unusually strong attachment to him. It's infuriating to think some man could claim his baby was "better bonded" just because when he bottle-fed her, the bottle was held in a ridiculous bib tied around his neck, rather than his hand. Since father, grandparent, baby-sitter or Jack the Ripper could feed the baby, one wonders whose "familiar voice" it might be to which the baby was supposed to bond. One wonders also if the child's mother might tie a replica of part of the male anatomy to herself to gain equality and further confuse the child.

Bottle-feeding is not equal to or interchangeable with breast-feeding, even though the formula companies would like us to think so. There's a vast difference between "breast-feeding" which is feeding milk from a breast instead of a bottle, and the loving method of nurturing a baby in what is truly "nursing," Someone who "nurses" another comforts them and helps them to do things they cannot do for themselves.

When you obtain breastfeeding information, check to see who supplied the information. If it's from a formula company, don't trust it. Think about it! Why would a formula company want you to breastfeed?

The formula company provides breastfeeding information so you think you can trust them. The message in their literature sounds that hopeful you breastfeed, but if you can't, they are there to help you. Isn't that nice? They appear to be the savior, providing the best nutrition for the mother who can't nurse her child.

So you won't feel bad about not breastfeeding, they try to make bottle-feeding equal to breastfeeding using the idiotic statement, "Breast is best, but bottle-feeding is just as good." Another trick is with the equation: Bottle-feeding + cuddling = breastfeeding.

These booklets are very carefully written. They contain some helpful breastfeeding information, but like the proverbial wolf in sheep's clothing, the good is merely covering over the subtle suggestions that you are going to need their product eventually. Like taking a little bit of toxin with your vegetables and whole grains, it poisons your mind with thoughts of failure.

One such booklet has a chart showing what a typical day is like with a new baby. It schedules your home to run like a factory, listing the number of hours and minutes the baby should sleep, the number of ounces of milk from breast-or-bottle at four-hour intervals, and recommends giving water between feedings. Try to follow it and you will be miserable, for it's a rare baby who actually will sleep for long periods of time, only waking up to nurse every four hours and go right back to sleep.

Some babies do, of course, and the parents of those babies wonder what the rest of us are complaining about. "This is easy!" They brag, "I just feed him and put him in his crib, and he falls asleep! I've got this business of baby care figured out!" Then they write a Baby Care book. Meanwhile, the rest of us are so busy rocking and carrying and nursing and nursing and nursing babies who never sleep, and reading Baby Care books for answers, we don't have time to write books.

Sometimes the wording implies breastfeeding is difficult, awkward, too tiring or even dangerous if the mother is sick. If you study these breastfeeding booklets carefully, the subliminal messages become quite obvious. For example, in one booklet I noticed only the photographs of bottle-feeding parents showed eye contact and smiling.

The formula companies produce lovely breastfeeding posters, too. One I noticed in a public health unit read "Breast milk is the best food for young infants." *Young infants*, the poster said. How long does an infant stay young? The inferred message is "Breast is best, but not for long." Furthermore, the message coldly tells us nursing the baby is nothing more than "food."

If it Aint Broke

Many women have trouble breastfeeding, or just plain old don't enjoy it because we have taken a simple, natural function and made it so darn complicated. How often should the child nurse? For how long? If the baby is fussing, is it because I ate strawberries? Will lack of sleep affect my milk supply? If he sleeps through a feeding, do I still use the last breast first? If he feeds 15 minutes on one breast and 6 minutes on the other, then sleeps two hours, should I multiply the number of minutes by the baby's birth weight and divide it by my bra size to get the square root of the problem?

Breastfeeding

Dr. Jack Newman, director of the Breastfeeding Clinic in Toronto, has compiled a list of breastfeeding myths he gives as a handout to nursing mothers at the clinic. He pokes fun at the notion of breastfeeding as the cause of all a mother's troubles:

> Family, health professionals, neighbours, friends and taxi drivers will blame the breastfeeding if the mother is tired, nervous, weepy, sick, has pain in her knees, has difficulty sleeping, is always sleeping, feels dizzy, is anemic, has a relapse of arthritis (migraines, or any chronic problem) complains of hair loss, change of vision, ringing in her ears or itchy skin. Breastfeeding will be blamed as the cause of marriage problems and the other children acting up. Breastfeeding is to blame when the mortgage rates go up and the economy is faltering. And whenever there is something that does not fit in with the "picture book" life, the mother will be advised by everyone that it will be better is she stops breastfeeding[16].

People usually agree with the statement "Breast is best," but this is an example of the so-called support a woman gets for doing the very best for her child.

Breastfeeding assures the baby spends the extra time wrapped up in his mother's arms, his soft skin against her breast, smelling her warm scent, hearing her heartbeat, feeling her movements. This is not only good for the baby, but good for the mother.

Some feminists would have us believe there is really no difference between men and woman other than what we have been socialized to believe. They are ignoring the obvious: Hormones.

Every time a woman breastfeeds her baby, the hormone *prolactin* pumps through her body. Prolactin is the mothering hormone, causing nurturing behavior. You can see this hormone in action. Suppose your dog just delivered her first litter of puppies and she's lying there looking a little bewildered. Not quite sure what to do, she sniffs at the pups and gets up and steps on them. You know what she needs to solve her puzzle: she needs to lie down and get the puppies nursing. Sure enough, once they start nursing, she seems to understand, and starts nuzzling her babies and licking them. Such behaviors are the effect of prolactin, the milk-making hormone.

Sometimes I have seen the hormone working when talking to a mother nursing her baby. In the middle of a conversation she suddenly looks down lovingly at her baby, caresses his little head, and forgets what she was talking about! The hormone relaxes you, and if you nurse the baby in bed, you can easily drift off into a blissful sleep with the baby.

Oxytocin, which causes the milk to move into the milk ducts, is recognized as the love hormone. God intended for us to have plenty of prolactin and oxytocin in our bloodstream when we have the overwhelming responsibility of caring for our babies. The hormones cause nurturing behaviors which mothering easier. We ought to pity the poor women who choose to bottle-feed and must cope with the demands of motherhood without the hormonal help.

The more you nurse, the more prolactin and oxytocin you have. Aha! Hormones! That explains why the women at the Leche League meeting who nurse more frequently seem to be the happier and less frustrated than the women who worked so hard at getting their babies on a four-hour schedules with no night feedings! La Leche League women were getting frequent boosts of mothering hormones.

"You don't need to keep track of how often you nurse the baby, any more than you keep track of how often you kiss the baby," La Leche League taught me. By watching the baby instead of the clock you soon recognize signals the baby gives to indicate he wants to nurse, long before he gets to the point of crying! You wouldn't wait until he is crying to feed him, any more than you would wait until you are cranky and lightheaded yourself before you eat. Instead, you become more aware of the non-verbal cues your baby uses: perhaps a facial grimace, rooting mouth movements or lip-smacking, restlessness and squirming which isn't just for a change of position. Others are amazed because your baby always seems so quiet and happy.

La Leche League helped me realize what made all the difference was simply attitude. We tend to focus on the negative aspects of nursing: Ugh, my breasts leak. My nipples are sore. I can't go anywhere without dragging the kid along. I have to stop and feed every two hours. I never get a full night's sleep. As mothers we need each other for support when the going gets rough and encouragement to go on. Isn't that how we do our best at any job?

Learn to accept the negative aspects of nursing in light of the joy we can experience too. We learn to appreciate and actually savour this precious time, enjoying the fullness of the unconditional love from your baby. Breastmilk is like love: the more you give away, the more you have to give.

Those tender moments of nursing when you feel the baby's whole body relax, give you a tremendous sense of satisfaction, knowing it was you alone who soothed your baby. You feel so special, so valuable. He melts into your arms and his eyes roll in utter ecstasy when your milk fills his tummy. He lets go of the breast and rolls back slightly, sighing like a satisfied lover, a drunken, glassy look in his eyes. Thus he falls asleep, in complete and total bliss, wrapped in your loving embrace.

A pox on the so-called expert who tells women they should never allow baby to fall asleep at the breast, calling this beautiful moment a "bad habit".

Prophylactation?

Nursing exclusively and frequently keeps your hormones at a high enough level to reduce your chance of conceiving another child until your body is ready. This really does work, if you follow God's plan of nursing your baby by the Golden Rule. Do unto your baby as you would have had your mother do unto you when you were a baby. The Golden Rule reads differently; maybe I should call it the Silver Rule, since it significantly summarizes the Simple Secrets for Successful Suckling.

We all know someone who got pregnant while they were nursing. It annoys me when someone who gives birth every 11 months claims it is God's will but they haven't practiced God's will for feeding the baby. The Almighty did not send a schedule and a stopwatch with the afterbirth, but He did give babies a heart-piercing cry and He made them unbearably cute for a reason. If you nurse the unbearably cute baby often enough he doesn't have to use his heart-piercing cry, you get rewarded with high levels of the mothering hormone and the love hormone, a happy, thriving baby who rarely cries, and unlimited conception-free sex for several months. According to Sheila Kippley, in *Breastfeeding and Natural Child Spacing*, the average length of time for nursing women to remain infertile is 14.6 months.[i]

Another seldom-cited benefit of breastfeeding is the reduced risk chances of developing breast cancer. Generations of women were discouraged from lactating, being told of the man-made methods of modern infant feeding were superior to the old-fashioned way. However, "There is a way that seemeth right unto a man, but the end thereof are the ways of death[ii]," for breast cancer is now the number two leading cause of cancer deaths in North American women. By simply using our breasts in the way the Good Lord intended, we prevent breast cancer, prevent pregnancy and prevent anemia since we aren't losing blood through menstruation. Thank God for the prophylactic benefits of lactation. Amen.

A Lifetime of Lessons Learned

The close relationship between a mother and child through breastfeeding has a profound impact on a child's future. Unfortunately this important is often overlooked in a society demanding universal daycare for all. Life's most important lessons

---

[i] This average applies to women using unrestricted breastfeeding. Many women go two years or more without menstruating.

[ii] Proverbs 14:12

absorbed in those early years, as we learned from Robert Fulgrum's *Everything I need to Learn about Life, I Learned in Kindergarten.* Where does one learn lifetime commitment but by example? For when the child sees his mother committed to him, day after day — even when she doesn't feel like it; (for better or worse) even if she could afford the best nanny and the best formula in the country; (for richer or poorer), even when she is ill; (in sickness and in health) even when she wants to go to a party or must attend funeral and doesn't want to be burdened with a baby; (in joy and in sorrow) — that is when he learns to love, honour, and obey.

How Successful Breastfeeding Is Related to Successful Birthing

When I first learned of La Leche League's recommendation to be awake and aware and an active participant in the birth, I wondered why the birth would have anything to do with breastfeeding. It turns out there are many reasons. Medications have a negative effect on your hormones. In the normal process of un-medicated birth, adrenaline pumps through your system. This helps makes the baby alert and able to bond with you as soon as he's born. Endorphins released during are natural painkillers and are what provide you the emotional high after delivery. Your confidence in yourself is heightened, including your ability to care for your baby.

Even though I had not been able to give birth, what I learned about breastfeeding – both by reading and through experience – helped build self–esteem and confidence in my body's ability to do what it was designed to do. I believed that by applying the principles of successful breastfeeding to childbirth, I learned to give birth easily, naturally, and joyfully.

- Sometimes, you simply hate breastfeeding. It's too tiring and you want to give up. Some understanding support from a woman who's been through the daunting times will encourage you to continue and help you get through the low times. *Likewise, sometimes labour is too hard and you wish you had had an epidural / a cesarean / your tubes tied. Encouragement from another woman who understands and supports you can help you through the difficult parts!*
- Rules and limitations on breastfeeding cause unnecessary stress. They take the focus off the baby and onto the clock. It harms the building relationship. Relax, forget the rules and accept the baby as an individual. *Likewise, rules and limitations on labour cause unnecessary stress. Focus on the coming baby, not the number of hours passed or the number of centimetres reached. Relax and accept the uniqueness of this labour.*

Breastfeeding

- The happily nursing mother feels pleased with her accomplishment as the baby grows on nothing but her milk. Watching her baby thrive on milk from her own body builds her self-esteem. She doesn't need any man-made formula or bottles when she already makes the best! *Likewise when childbirth is done by the mother, not to the mother, it is empowering. It is she who gives birth, she has the power, and she pushes the baby out. She doesn't need any man-made objects to pull it out for her.*
- Hormones released while breastfeeding have a calming effect and help the mother feeling loving toward her baby. The more she nurses, the more hormones are released. In this symbiotic relationship, caring for the baby is a loving act no more difficult for the mother than caring for herself. *Likewise, hormones released when in labour are good for both mother and baby: Endorphins are natural pain-killers, provide an emotional "high," and enhance bonding behaviour. Adrenaline puts mother in a highly aware state and makes baby alert and able to bond. We shouldn't mess with the natural hormonal state.*
- Baby is an equal partner in the nursing relationship. You work together: he indicates his need, and you respond. He regulates the amount according to need. You can't over-feed him. *Likewise, baby will come in his own time. You can't hurry it; you can only accept it. The time to push is when it feels right to push.*
- Breastfeeding is so beautiful: God designed it, it works, and I trust it. Breastfeeding prevents conception. Without me having to do a thing, my milk changes in volume, consistency and taste. The hormones help me be a calm mother. *God also designed childbirth. I trust it will work even without interference. I know all things work together for good even when they don't seem to make sense at first.*
- As the baby's mother, I know more about him than anybody else. I'm the one who can tell when he wants to nurse when no one else would notice. It teaches me to trust my instinct. *I also know my body better than the doctor. My body knows what it needs, too, better than the doctor. I trust what my body will tell me to do in labour, whether it's to walk, sit, dance, squat, or lie on my side.*
- FEAR and WORRY have a negative effect on breastfeeding. They inhibit the mother's natural response to her child. It's harder for the milk to let down when under a lot of stress. *FEAR and WORRY also have a negative effect on labour. Fear can cause the body to release too much adrenaline in a fight-or-flight response, shutting down the birthing hormones.*

- Even those who seem to be supportive of breastfeeding may secretly want you to fail. Formula companies distribute not-so-helpful books pretending to help you breastfeed, when they'd really prefer you purchased their product instead. Even friends or relatives may secretly hope to see you fail if they feel guilty for not nursing their own children. E*ven though the doctor claims to be in favor of natural childbirth, it's better for him if he has control over the time and place and method of delivery. Financially it's better for him if I have a cesarean, especially if he can do it at a pre-arranged time. Even friends or family may feel cheated or jealous to see me experience something they have missed.*
- Doctors don't know near as much about breastfeeding as women who have successfully breastfed. Many of their suggestions are detrimental to the natural course of breastfeeding and actually cause breastfeeding failure. *Likewise, my doctor has never given birth. He doesn't know what it feels like, and can offer me little more than drugs to help me cope with labour. Some of the things he recommends are in fact detrimental to natural labour and delivery, and actually cause failure to progress.*
- Breastfeeding is related to other aspects of female sexuality: it is aided by an un-medicated birth, prevents conception, and affects libido. *A positive birth experience is likewise going to affect other aspects of female sexuality.*
- Nursing isn't just the "noble" thing to do, but can be wonderfully enjoyable for the mother. It can make her feel good. It can be very sensuous. Not sensuous like an orgasm, but sensuous like a good backrub. *Perhaps giving birth can also be something wonderful... a time for couples to work together lovingly to complete the act which was started at conception.*

CHAPTER 5

VBAC – Vaginal Birth After Cesarean

"Do I bring to the moment of birth and not give delivery?" says the Lord. "Do I close up the womb when I bring to delivery?" says your God.

- Isaiah 66:9

The road map for the journey to my VBAC started with the book Silent Knife: Cesarean Prevention and Vaginal Birth After Cesarean by Lois J. Estner and Nancy Wainer Cohen. It is the most comprehensive book about how to avoid unnatural childbirth I have ever read. It's much better than the book you're reading now. If you are planning a VBAC throw this one away and go get Silent Knife. In it you will find well-documented research into the safety of VBAC, detailed lists of the often-surprising interventions which can lead to cesareans, and countless personal stories of women who have been victims of unnecessary cesarean sections, as well as those who have braved the VBAC experience. It was my VBAC bible. I could hardly get through the book the first time I read it because I would so often be in tears as I read the stories from other women who had had cesareans, and were also suffering. What a relief it was to read accounts from those who know how it hurts to have missed the baby's birth and felt like they have been cheated.

After reading Silent Knife and realizing my emotional response was normal, I allowed myself to wallow in self-pity for the first time, crying on the shoulder of a new friend who I discovered was equally traumatized by her cesarean. She was the only person I knew who really understood how I felt. We could confide our deepest hurt to each other without reprimand.

VBAC

Once the grieving was fulfilled, I was free to move on. I became angry. Angry with the doctors, the nurses, the hospitals, the whole system that treats childbirth like a disease that must be cured. I believe such anger is healthy, because anger motivates people to action. The alternative is helplessness and a resignation to succumb to the demands of the medical system once again, needlessly placing your life, your dignity, and your baby in their hands.

Armed with the carefully researched information gleaned from Silent Knife, I made an appointment to speak to the obstetrician who had done my cesarean. I wanted to hear directly from his lips why I needed a C/section. What was wrong with my body? Would I be able to have a VBAC? Under what conditions? And what percentage of his patients actually did achieve a VBAC?

We had a long talk. He told me, (get this:) "Your failure to progress in labour is Nature's way of telling us your pelvis was too small to deliver this baby." *Nature's way? This is what he considers working with Nature?*

Dr. N said I might be able to have a vaginal birth if — and only if — I followed his instructions very carefully: As his patient, I would not be allowed to gain more than twenty pounds. I would be permitted to go up to my due date, but not past it. I would be required to go to the hospital immediately at the first hint of labour at which time I would be put straight to bed and have an IV inserted. Then my membranes would be ruptured so an internal fetal monitor could be attached. Of course the monitor requires the patient to remain motionless. I would be permitted to labour for up to twelve hours of labour but no more, lest I put "too much stress on the scar." If labour lasted longer than the allotted twelve hours, I'd be induced. Under those regulations, and only if the baby was assessed to weigh less than 7 pounds, he thought I might be able to deliver vaginally. Maybe a 30% chance, he said. Then, immediately after the delivery of the placenta Dr. N would do a "manual exploration" of the uterus, meaning he would put his entire hand up inside of me and feel around for any holes to make sure the scar was still intact.

"You can still have the baby 'natural,' if you want," he added.

Natural? *NATURAL?* What was "natural" about any of those things he planned on doing to me? "Natural" to him meant simply un-medicated. What woman in her right mind would submit to such torture without being drugged?

What is so natural about being restrained in a bed flat on your back when you're in labour? What is so natural about having the membranes ruptured with a hook? Is it natural to have an IV in my arm and a catheter in my bladder? How natural is the labouring process when hormones are being pumped into the bloodstream to induce stronger uterine contractions? How natural is the 12-hour limit? And worst of all, how natural is it to become a human hand puppet by his "manual exploration"?! How could Dr. N know anything about "Natural" when he has likely never seen a truly natural, uninhibited birth? He obviously did not even trust nature.

At this point I brought up some of the statistics I had memorized from Silent Knife in the chapter on Uterine Dependability and fired questions at him.

"Isn't there a higher risk of uterine rupture from induction than there is from VBAC?" I asked.

"What about the increased risk of infection with ruptured membranes?

"Isn't it true labour progresses faster when the woman is up walking than when she's lying in bed?

"Isn't there a higher risk of fetal distress from being flat on my back?

"What about the possibility of introducing infection by doing a manual exploration of the uterus?"

He asked suspiciously where I obtained this information.

"The statistics are from the National Institute of Health. I read it in Silent Knife." He had never heard of the book, of course. I asked him if he would like to read it.

"No," he answered angrily, "Would you like to read *William's Obstetrics*?"

"I have."

He was insulted by my questions which I can certainly understand. It took a lot of years of school and experience for him to get where he was only to have some dumb housewife question his procedures. But the statistics *were* all correct. There were risks involved either way. The doctor chose to take admittedly greater risks because it would give him more control over the labour and delivery. I preferred to take the statistically safer, more natural approach, but the responsibility would fall upon me.

Dr. N then ended the interview, saying he would be happy to allow me a trial of labour with my next baby, and to call him when I got pregnant. I shook his uterus-exploring hand goodbye, and smiling sweetly said, "I am already three months pregnant, and there's no way you will deliver this baby."

But as soon as I left his office I began to worry about what I had just done. *Now what am I going to do?* I worried. What if no other doctor would take my case? What if I had to have another cesarean and ended up with him anyway? And what if he did something mean like keep my baby in the ICU to teach me a lesson after what I said? (See I'm just as scared as you are!)

I knew I was being ridiculous. Surely someone somewhere could deliver this baby without treating me like an explosive uterus. I started hunting for another doctor and kept running into the same thing. Most of them agreed to let me attempt a "Trial of Labour," but at this trial my uterus would be considered guilty until proven innocent. The doctors always implied I was choosing a "nice experience" over my baby's safety, and what kind of a mother would do such a thing?

At a La Leche League Conference I made some connections with other women who had actually *had* a VBAC. A few of us decided to get together and have some meetings, La Leche League style. We'd offer information, encouragement and support. We'd discuss our cesareans and VBAC experiences in order to achieve our VBAC goals.

I got in contact with a midwife who lived not too far from me and met with her. Tall and slender, soft-spoken Elana had a calm confidence about her. Always immaculately dressed, she emanated professionalism. I decided to hire her for the birth. This was 1985, and the government did not yet recognize midwives as legal practitioners. Contrary to what most people thought, this did not mean midwives were illegal; it just meant they were not recognized as a profession. She had delivered many babies at home, but her role within the hospital could only be recognized as a Labour Assistant. I also found a doctor who was trained in the Netherlands where homebirth is quite common, and did not think a previous cesarean was a major risk factor. It was not a big deal in the Old Country, Dr. Oosterhuis said. However, because it is risky according to North American medical protocol, I had to meet with an obstetrician for assessment during my pregnancy who gave me the same "Trial of Labour" rules and limitations. Dr. Oosterhuis said not to worry, I was *his* patient, and he didn't see any reason we'd require an obstetrician since I was healthy and everything appeared to be fine. Unlike the OB, he seemed to expect the best during birth, not the worst. His positive attitude was infectious and I left his office feeling much more confident about having a natural birth.

Throughout my second pregnancy I made every effort to make sure there were no stumbling blocks for a VBAC. I enjoyed excellent nutrition: no alcohol, tea, or coffee; no white flour or sugar. I got plenty of rest and exercise and was still riding my bicycle past my due date. I went to the chiropractor regularly. I took vitamins and drank raspberry-leaf tea. I read everything I could find about VBAC, pregnancy, nutrition, and natural childbirth. I reread Silent Knife and cried again. I tried to think positive thoughts about the birth and visualize myself actually doing it. I had a lot of strange dreams, though. I remember one for instance, in which there was a baby in an oven. The oven was getting hot and I couldn't get the baby out, couldn't reach it no matter what I did. It was obviously a dream about my cesarean. I lay in bed thinking about my unfinished dream until I made sure I found a way to get the baby out of the oven – by myself.

I tried to avoid negative comments, but I sure got them! I was called crazy and "fanatical." I was accused of being selfish for wanting a good birth more than a healthy baby, as if a normal birth would risk my baby's life. Many people assumed I'd already have my surgery booked and wanted to know what day the baby was coming. To avoid the inevitable questions I simply answered a non-committal, "We'll see what happens when the time comes," and changed the subject.

I took more control over my health care, even with petty things. I refused a pregnancy test, for instance. I knew I was pregnant, I knew when I conceived, I recognized the changes in my body, and I knew when I was due, so why waste time and money on a pregnancy test? I altered the regular schedule of doctor visits to suit *me* better. I considered it another waste of my time and money to make a trip to the doctor's office every month just to have him weigh me and take my blood pressure. While some may consider this to be irresponsible, I found the opposite to be true. It forced me to be more aware of my own body, paying attention to slight physical changes, instead of relying on the doctor to notice any abnormality.

Each time I visited the doctor, I would also go to the midwife for prenatal visits. Both places recorded my weight, blood pressure, and fundal height (the top of the uterus); both people would check the baby's position and listen to the heart tones. But there was a remarkable contrast between the appointments.

Elana's prenatal clinics were held in her own home. There were often other pregnant moms there for their appointments, new babies for postpartum visits and toddlers with their parents. Many clients would bring Elana a loaf of banana bread or some homemade cookies, and there was always a pot of herbal tea made. Sometimes women would visit over tea while waiting for their turn, washing up their cups and plates before they left.

At the doctor's office, the nurse would ask me for a urine sample and she would weigh me. Elana would point me to the bathroom to weigh myself and test my own urine. It's not hard to do. You don't need medical training to pee on a plastic stick and match the colour to the chart on the dipstick bottle. My blood pressure was often a little higher at the doctor's office. This is not uncommon, and even has a name: White Coat Hypertension. Many patients have a higher blood pressure just because of the stress of being at the doctor's office.

Elana's visits took longer than the doctor's did because she would talk about my family, my fears, and my preparation for the upcoming birth. She had several birth videos you could watch on her TV and a library of interesting birth books to borrow. And she always made a point to ask me about my diet, and would righteously nag at me if I weren't eating enough fruits and vegetables.

Throughout the pregnancy, however, my husband was NOT supportive. He believed the doctor had rescued our baby from my body and was scared that I would hurt our baby if I attempted to squeeze it through my "small pelvis." It was very stressful for him as well as for me to be planning for a VBAC. It would have been easier for everyone - for Bert, for the doctor and the obstetrician, and for my own anxiety - to simply plan a cesarean section. We'd know weeks in advance the day our baby would be delivered and be prepared for it. My only support came from my midwife, Dr. Oosterhuis, and friends who are natural childbirth advocates.

One surprising thing which changed Bert's mind occurred when I dragged him to a VBAC meeting. (We had arranged a special meeting for the daddies to come to, each of us lying, "All the *other* husbands are going!") I noticed Bert chatting with one of the other men whose wife had had a VBAC. After the meeting Bert seemed more relaxed and agreed VBAC was at least a possibility. I wanted to know what John had said to convince Bert VBAC was a safe option and well worth the effort. It turned out they had been talking about playing hockey! But as Bert saw it: if a normal down-to-earth, hockey-playing, beer-drinking, every-day-type-guy like John could handle VBAC, he could too!

Labour Day (and-a-half)

Six days past my due date on a warm, beautiful day in late spring I started feeling some contractions, a bit different than the Braxton-Hicks I had felt for several weeks. I didn't even mention anything to my mother when I went to visit her, even though my back was sore and I put one foot on a stool as we chatted and cleaned the fresh-picked strawberries. At suppertime I called my midwife to let her know about the mild labour pains, but found she had broken her foot and was in the hospital! But, devoted as she was, she said as soon as they let her out of the ER she would come, if we could pick her up.

It was about 11:00 at night when we got home, carried sleeping Joshua up to bed and got the midwife to check me. Since I was only 3 cm dilated, she lay down on the couch with her foot on ice, and everyone went to bed to rest while we still could. I couldn't. I had to move my legs during contractions because my back was hurting so I got up to walk around. At midnight I called my best friend Terry to tell her this was it! She was also expecting her second baby and was also planning a VBAC so she was very excited for me. She made me promise to keep her in touch no matter what the hour. She'd keep the phone by her pillow and pray for me.

I start pacing the floor. During contractions, I lean my hands on a wall and do a funny waltz to rock my pelvis. I have to keep moving, can't keep my legs still. Elana suggests I take a hot bath to see if it helps. It doesn't. I notice a bloody show, and remember the dress I'm wearing is borrowed, perhaps I should change. I decide to keep wearing it because I love the way it feels - a loose, flowing sundress. I want to be loose, I want to be pretty.

3:30 am. I phone Terry. "This HURTS!" I tell her. She offers some suggestions: Have you tried taking calcium? Vitamin E? Raspberry Leaf tea? Yes, dammit, but it's not helping much. I try another hot bath; I get out and pace some more and rock, rock, rock my pelvis. Is this normal? Normal for you, Elana says.

4:30 am. Oh, my back hurts. I have Bert call my mother to come over. I'll have to leave soon and she's going to be watching Joshua while we're in the hospital. I'm only five centimetres.

5:30 am. The sun is rising already and I'm tired. Mom fetches a pillow and blanket and I lie on the floor on my side, dozing off between contractions. She kneels behind me and rubs my back when she notices a contraction starting. It helps. She's a mother, and she knows where it hurts.

7:30 am. I'm getting tired of this and frustrated. I get in the tub again for the fourth time, but it doesn't help. It feels better when I can lean on someone. I put one arm around Bert's neck and one around my mother, taking the weight off my lower body. Six centimeters...that's where I got stuck last time. I want to go to the hospital now, before this gets worse and I have to sit still in a car.

One more call to Terry before we go. "Did you talk me into this?" I complain, half joking, "I'm dying and nobody believes me!" She makes me laugh and encourages me. I wish she could come over.

It's a torturous half-hour drive; every little bump magnified tenfold in my uterus. We stop and buy a soft drink for me. "They may not allow you anything to eat or drink once you get to the hospital," the midwife says, "and the sugar will do you good at this point."

At the hospital they bring me a wheelchair. They've got to be kidding! My back is killing me; I can't sit! Policy states they must at least follow me with the wheelchair. Down the hall and up the elevator they follow me with the wheelchair at my backside, like they expect me to fall over. I hold the railing and rock my pelvis in the elevator.

The labour room is a small, ugly green room. A fetal monitor sits next to the bed looking like something from Star Wars. I want R2D2 out of there so there will be room to pace around the bed and over Elana's crutches. The nurse brings in a Patient Uniform for me and forms to sign and asks a bunch of questions I cannot comprehend when my brain is in my uterus. Thank goodness Elana can help with some of it. I politely decline, again and again, the nurse's suggestion I wear the hospital Patient Uniform. No thank-you. She's afraid mine might get soiled. I picked it out especially for this occasion and I don't care if it gets dirty.

The intern and the resident come in. We lie, telling them I've only been in labour about eight hours. One of them, I am told, must do an internal. Which one would I prefer? I look down at their hands and pick the woman - she has smaller fingers!

As soon as they find out the previous birth was a cesarean section, they call the obstetrician. I wish my own doctor would get here, so everyone else will leave me alone.

I dread the thought of the internal because it means lying on the bed. I need to keep walking; it hurts too much to be still. "Hurry up," I snap. The resident or intern or whatever she is cannot reach my cervix with her small fingers, and shoves her hand, ramming her fist against my perineum, pushing against those sensitive tissues. Like a scene from The Exorcist, I suddenly spew forth language which leaves everyone in the room blushing. "How could you DO that?!" I continue to scream at her, "What are you going to do next, take a run at it? You're a woman! Don't you know how much it HURTS?" (I get a little cranky when I'm in labour, apparently.)

9:30 am. Finally my doctor arrives, thank God! All the staff members seem to relax, knowing this VBAC is his responsibility, so the resident, intern, and nurses leave us alone. I'm pacing around the tiny room, tripping over Elana's crutches, back aching, hips aching. I wrap one arm around Bert's neck and one around Dr. O's, suspending my weight on their shoulders. Dr. Oosterhuis doesn't seem to mind. I feel a little foolish, but it hurts less in my hips and back this way.

He decides it's time to check me, so I reluctantly climb on the bed as soon as the contraction is over. I tell him to make it quick so I can be on my feet before the next contraction hits. As he examines me, my water breaks with a gush across the bed and I begin to shake violently. Suddenly the contraction hits like a tidal wave, knocking me over, leaving me gasping, and I let out a loud holler which likely frightens everyone on the ward. I grab Bert's hands and squeeze with all my might, moaning, yelling Elana, rub my back! Ohhh!

I remember! This must be what they call transition! Another wave crashes over me and I holler and cry out in pain once more. It's agony; I can't stand the pain. How much longer? I can't take it!

Dr. Oosterhuis says the baby is up pretty high still, so knowing gravity will help move the baby down, I get off the bed. Once I'm up, I can handle the pain again. Someone mentions I should be heading to the delivery room so I start walking there. I look back and see I am the leader in a comic parade: Bert and Dr. O are both rushing to put on their operating-room greens, hopping on one foot, each of them jumping as they pull up their pants to chase me down the corridor. Elana trails behind, leaning on her crutches while she pulls on her paper cap, also trying to catch up to me as I waddle down the hall. The open-mouthed nurses observe the procession from the sidelines, incredulous. "She's walking to the delivery room? Nobody walks to the delivery room!"

To my surprise, I find the delivery room looks just like an operating room. I expected it would have a bed in it like the birthing room next door where I had laboured two years earlier. The delivery table is just that: a table. I anticipated at least a backrest or something. Who wants to give birth on a TABLE? They get me into position and the doctor pokes inside me to push a rim of the cervix back. OUCH!! Now, push, they say.

I can't push, it HURTS! What about the wonderful urge to push I've heard about? I try to fake pushing; making a few token grunts, but nobody is fooled. I try pushing on my left side, on my right side, then on my hands and knees on the delivery table, naked butt in the air like a porno star.... Nothing.

So I get off the table and pace around the delivery room, round and round the table, under the bright lights, past all the frightening shiny equipment, neatly displayed and ready for me. Two nurses, the small-fingered resident and intern, Bert, Elana, and Doctor O and maybe more, all sit on their stools, or stand watching, their eyes following my every move. They're all masked and gowned; I'm in bare feet in my sexy little blue nightgown. It's like being in an alien spaceship, the object of some strange experiment.

I pace around and around the room, crowded enough with people, let alone the monitor, the IV pole, the equipment tables, the incubator and whatever other machines are there. Motioning for Bert to come to me, I put my arms around his neck and push, standing up, closing my eyes to block out the staring eyes. I can tell by the looks on the faces of the staff, this is highly unusual.

I put my back to Bert and squat, supported by him with his hands under my arms. I arch my back and push. It seems to be working, but one nurse tells me I'm doing it all wrong. You don't arch back, she instructs, you must curl forward to push properly.

They keep warning me I have to get back on the table when I feel rectal pressure. Well, I feel it, but I'm not telling! I know darn well the baby isn't going to fall out on the floor without me noticing! Push! Push! More! Harder! They keep yelling at me. Damn, I wish they'd leave me alone. I don't feel like pushing; there is no urge to do so.

Because of their incessant nagging I get back on the delivery table. I'm just so darn uncomfortable no matter what position I try, I give up and lie on the table in <u>*their*</u> *favorite position: on my back with my legs in the stirrups.*

Elana whispers to me. "You HAVE to push." she says, leaning over her crutches, "They won't give you a lot of time. They're getting ready to label this a 'Failure to Progress'."

I picture the obstetrician standing outside the delivery room door, sharpening his scalpel and laughing an evil laugh, dollar signs in his eyes. So I PUSH! I push and push with all my might until the contraction ends.

A minute's rest, then someone whose hand is on my belly tells Bert another contraction is coming. He pushes my pillow forward to help me into a more upright position. I take a deep breath and push, straining until my ears are hissing, blocking out all else. I can feel my face getting red and hot, and the pressure in my head is like a balloon about to burst. The contraction ends and I flop back, exhausted. Again. Again.

Flat out, except the legs still up in stirrups, I am surprised to find myself sound asleep between contractions. I glance at the clock. I've been pushing over an hour. Doctor K was right I think, I must have an androgenous pelvis. I envision my pelvis is shaped like a funnel, each push squeezing the baby, wedging it in, crushing its little skull.

It hurts so bad to push and there is no urge to push. I swear at the doctor, telling him he's hurting me. Everyone in the room is yelling at me. PUSH! PUSH! PUSH! Some sound like encouraging words, but some sound like a football coach, aiming to get the players mad enough to be more aggressive. I hate them all, every one of them. I am in hell, and these are my tormentors. They won't let me rest; they torture me with pain and their shouts and this will go on for all eternity because I'm bad and evil and I deserve this torture for wanting a VBAC, for putting my baby through this just because of my own selfish desire for birth.

Doctor O is sitting on the stool between my legs, JUST SITTING THERE, with his arms folded across his chest. "Get the forceps!" I yell at him, and he ignores me. It's useless. Oh, it hurts. Is it supposed to hurt this bad? Maybe it hurts so badly because my uterus has ruptured. Why didn't I just book a cesarean when I had the chance? I could have had a c-section two weeks ago, and I'd be at home with my baby right now. I wouldn't be suffering like this.

"Your baby has dark hair," Dr. O says when the contraction ends. I don't know what he's talking about. What baby? He clips a piece of hair and hands it to me to prove it. He must be mistaken, I think. Idiot, he must have clipped some of my pubic hair, thinking it was a baby's head. There's no baby.

This pain, this VBAC is useless. I'm sure I've ruptured because it hurts so badly. If I've ruptured, I am hemorrhaging, so I might as well get this baby out. It'll be dead anyway, and they'll have to start working on saving my life, before I bleed to death from the rupture. It's 1:00 and I've been pushing like this for two hours.

The nurse tells me I will soon feel a burning sensation. This "burning sensation" or "tingling" as I'd heard it described, occurred with the next contraction. Tingling? It was like a burning red-hot poker, pulling, stretching my skin beyond its limit. It was awful, fiery and it didn't go away with the contraction. I could see the alarmed expressions on the intern's faces, like they're thinking, "Isn't he going to DO something?" Dr. O picked up the scissors — and then dropped them on the floor! I think he did it on purpose. I reached down and felt a huge bulge where I should have felt my vagina. With my hands I gently tried to ease my stretched skin back, over this bulge to relieve the horrid stinging pain. Another highly unusual situation I can see from their expressions: a patient being allowed to touch herself? Now I have an urge to push, but only to get rid of this burning Ring of Fire!

One more push, and — Oh, some relief! But then I feel the doctor doing something — he's helping the shoulders out — and I feel movement inside of me, and Elana excitedly tells me Sheila, open your eyes, LOOK! LOOK! And I see a baby, a <u>real baby</u> being lifted to my tummy!

"It's a boy!" I squeal, and he opens his eyes and lets out a gurgling cry as he takes his first breath. He's purple and slippery-wet and he's just so beautiful the tears are streaming down my face. "Oh, Bert, look at him! We DID it! A baby boy!"

Dr. O believes the father should be the one to cut the cord and Bert does so, separating us. I love everyone in the room, and I never loved Bert so much as this moment...

Nobody takes the baby from me, another unusual situation. He stays in my arms until I finally ask them to find out what he weighs. Ten pounds, one and a half ounces! I am triumphant!

I had a small tear, which was why the burning was so bad. Dr. O said he wouldn't stitch it, just let it heal on its own. The raw open skin burned like a cigarette burn every time I urinated, so I took a jug of warm water with me to the toilet, to pour over myself while peeing. I put Vitamin E on the raw spot, too. It was healed completely within 6 days, a lot faster than most episiotomies heal. There was no pain when we resumed intercourse four weeks after the birth.

My son Clayton is the only person I know who had a haircut before he was born!

VBAC Recovery

The next morning, I was up and dressed and ready to go home before the 7:00 a.m. shift change. I would have gone home a few hours after the birth but they insisted I was bleeding a lot and made me stay. It was only the tear bleeding, nothing serious and no stitches were required.

"Are you sure you want to leave so soon?" the nurses asked, "We think you should stay another day. You're quite swollen 'down there'."

"So what?" I said, "I'm not sick, I'm just a little swollen. There's nothing you are doing for me here that can' at home." The only "treatment" was to have a sitz bath to promote healing of the tear. I'd sooner sitz in my own bath at home.

"There's Mommy!" Josh happily cried when he spotted me in the hospital corridor. It was the first night I had ever spent away from my little boy and I missed him. He ran to me, his arms open wide, and I scooped him up in a big bear hug. It felt so good. If I'd had a cesarean, I would still be in bed and on painkillers. I would not be able to allow my little boy on my lap, nor would I have been able to pick him up for weeks. How hard it would have been for him, not only dealing with my absence, but what he would consider in his two-year-old mind to be rejection.

An hour later as we pulled into the driveway with our new baby, it suddenly occurred to me how very simple childbirth was. Not easy, because it had been painful and exhausting, but simple because it was so *uncomplicated.* Twenty-four hours earlier, I had left the driveway in hard labour. Now I had returned to the same driveway, back to normal, only the baby was outside of me, not inside. There had not been any surgery from which I'd have to recover. There were no drugs to make birth occur, no IV, no stitches, and no monitor. There was nothing magic in the hospital to make the baby get born. It was difficult, but it was not mysterious. And it was me who did the difficult part. Me! Not the doctor, not the nurses, me! I was the only one who got the baby from the inside to the outside. The doctor just caught him.

My neighbour saw us pulling into the driveway and came running over, amazed to see me home so soon. Bert made some coffee and we sat and visited in the kitchen — in my own kitchen — just like always, except for the newborn baby in my arms. It was just so wonderfully normal! A friend called to find out what hospital I was in and was astonished when I answered the phone. *This is fun,* I thought, *I feel like a celebrity*!

Lessons from Birth #2

- Childbirth hurts. It was NOT an easy birth.
- The baby had been in a posterior position throughout labour, hence the backache. My crazy labour-dance, the Elvis-Pelvis Rock-Rock-Rock around the clock, and pushing with my back arched instead of curled, *was what turned the baby.*
- Apparently, I get a little cranky in labour.
- Holding one's wife, supporting her in your arms while she gives birth to your child has an impact on a man. It forces him to understand the depth of what is happening to the family. It's a far cry from waiting in the smoking room to hear from a stranger you have just become a father.
- There is something very sensual about giving birth. Nobody had told me about this! It occurred to me the moment I touched the hot, sticky-wet flesh when he was born, this was somehow very sexy. I hadn't figured it out yet, but I know something happened, and I got a glimpse of a deep, hidden secret at that moment.

CHAPTER 6

Letters from Kay

Modern Medicine is neither an art nor a science. It is a religion.

-Dr. Roberts S. Mendelsohn, MD

Dear Sheila

Can you help me?

I got your name from a friend. She said you had a cesarean, but have since had a couple of VBACs, even at home. She said you might be able to help.

I had a cesarean about a year ago, and I still have a hard time dealing with it. People who had normal births don't seem to understand what I am going through. They think I am being ridiculous if I mention how unhappy I was to have a cesarean. I am happy about having a healthy baby of course, but I feel like it's all an act: I smile and act happy even though I still feel so empty. I know I shouldn't feel this way, and I feel just terrible about it bothering me because I do have a healthy child. I guess that's the important thing.

Did you go through any of this, after your cesarean? How long does it take for the hurt to go away?

Sincerely,
Kay

Dear Kay

Does it help at all to know you are normal?

Some women don't give a hoot where the baby comes out of—it could be their ears for all they care. I doubt if your doctor cares much where the baby comes out either, or your husband for that matter. But it mattered to me and it mattered to you! I'm no psychiatrist, but I suspect grief after a cesarean is affected by several factors:

1. Were you hoping to have a natural childbirth? You are more likely to be very disappointed than the mother who said, "Just make sure I have no pain, or I'll sue!"
2. Did you consider cesarean as an option? Was there any possibility, any problem you could foresee prior to the delivery, or was it a complete surprise?
3. Was there an absolute reason for your section - an obvious immediate emergency such as a prolapsed cord or placenta previa, for which you are grateful? Or is there some question as to whether or not the cesarean was truly necessary?
4. If it was not an obvious emergency, did you feel you had any choice in the matter? Were other options explained to you, and the decision left up to you and your husband? Or were you led to believe the decision to do the surgery was out of your control?
5. How well did you recover physically? Did you have help at home during your recovery period?
6. Have you had a previous vaginal birth, so you know your body *can* work the way it's supposed to?
7. Were you conscious during the cesarean, so you remember the moment of birth, or did you wake up to find out it had already happened?

Giving birth was an experience you were looking forward to which you didn't get. I understand your unhappiness. Painful or not, you wanted to know what it was like to push a new baby into the world. Sharing such an experience unites you with millions of women around the world today and throughout history. Giving birth is a rite of passage into the New World of parenthood, and a sign of our womanliness.

It's hard to explain to those who don't understand why you feel a strange sense of loss. After all the planning and months of looking forward to this wonderful experience, you wake up and you've missed it. It's like missing out on Christmas or a graduation ceremony. Sure, you still have a baby, but you're too sore from the surgery to enjoy it.

Do you ever get up early on a summer morning to watch the sun rise? Experiencing the awesome changing colours blending the dark of night into the dawn of a new day is indescribable. But for the cesarean mom who missed the birth of her baby, her memory of the sunrise is nothing but a black and white photo.

But it's even worse than simple disappointment: giving birth is an expression of womanhood, so to miss the birth of the baby is like missing the conception. (Hey honey, guess what I did while you were asleep?) You were unconscious at one of the most profound moments of your life, the moment when you became a mother. You're left with an emptiness that's hard to describe.

How long does it take the hurt to go away? A year or more, for many women. Until you have a vaginal birth, for some. It helps to talk to someone who understands.

Hang in there, Kay, you're normal!

Sincerely,
Sheila

Dear Sheila

Thank you so much for writing! I feel like I can tell you this, and you won't think I am crazy!

For me, having a cesarean was not unlike being raped. Gang-raped in fact. Only this was legal!

I was often in tears after the birth, and everyone said it was just "Baby Blues," and perfectly normal. I assumed they were right; this is just what giving birth is like. One day when I was in tears again for no apparent reason, it suddenly hit me: I had been raped! Now it all made sense!

A man of high standing in the community committed this crime: my obstetrician. He had assured me he would do everything he could to help me have a natural childbirth experience, and I trusted him. But, once he had me in his territory, things were different.

The doctor/perpetrator and his gang (of students) confined me against my will. My private parts were exposed to - and fondled by - all of them. I was given drugs that would silence my protests, further immobilize me, and keep me quiet. They withheld food from me. The doctor had complete control over me, even threatening me with <u>death</u> (my baby's or my own) unless I cooperated with him. (He didn't threaten to kill me, of course, but terrified me by informing me what could happen to me or my baby in the worst case scenario.)

I was powerless and under his control, drugged and "tied" to the bed with tubes and wires and a monitor keeping track of my every move. So I let him have his way with me, sacrificing my body to him and his gang members to protect my baby.

When a woman is threatened and manipulated by a man who uses her sex organs for his own control and power, isn't it rape?

I also notice I have gone through the whole gamut of emotional turmoil, the same as rape victims do:

- FEAR came first, as they were preparing to do the surgery: Am I going to die? Is my baby going to die? What if I die but my baby lives? How will my husband cope? What if they cut me before I am asleep? What if they cut my baby?
- DAZED/CONFUSED When I came to - Where am I? What happened? Did I have a baby? Is it over? Where is my baby? Is my baby all right? Who are these people around me? Why do I hurt so much?
- DENIAL - I have a baby but how he got here doesn't matter. He's healthy, which is all that matters. What difference does it make how he was born? I tried to forget all about it.
- GUILT over my feelings of loss: A healthy baby should be all that matters, or at least everyone tells me so. I have no right to feel bad about this. How selfish I am.
- GUILT over what happened to the baby: My poor baby was pulled from my womb and I wasn't even awake to greet him. His daddy couldn't see him either. He was with strangers. How did he spend his first moments of life?
- WORRY - How do I really know for sure whether he *is* my baby? I was asleep when he was born. What if someone comes and claims him just as I start to fall in love with him?
- GUILT — over the cesarean: Why did I let them bully me? Why was I so weak? Maybe I was just selfish, wanting to escape the pain of childbirth. Did I do the right thing?
- GUILT – blaming myself: What did I do wrong? Why did this happen to me? Didn't I do as I was told, take good care of myself, swallow all my vitamins, and give up alcohol and caffeine and junk food? Didn't I go to all my prenatal visits and do everything the doctor said? Didn't I take all the classes to teach me everything? Didn't I practice my breathing exercises every night? What's wrong with my body? Why did I fail?
- DEPRESSION - My doctor saved the baby's life – saved him from me! I feel useless, perhaps even *dangerous*, to my baby. I feel ugly, inadequate. I have no purpose, no right to look after this child. This beautiful, innocent baby deserves better.

The worst thing was not being "there" when the baby was born. I was out of it for so many hours and didn't even see him until he was 7 hours old. I was the last to know I had had a baby boy. I know it sounds selfish but I thought I carried this child for nine months, went through all the pain, and I am the last to find out what he was and what he looked like. Somehow, it just didn't seem fair.

Thanks for "listening."

Kay

Dear Kay,

When I read your letter, the memories came flooding back to me. Marilyn Moran, author of Birth Pleasure says a typical childbirth in a typical medically-managed hospital birth is "Rape in Reverse:" Rape is the forceful invasion of the vagina, while a typical hospital delivery using episiotomy and forceps is the forceful evacuation of it. Both are equally traumatic experiences. No wonder so many women go through such debilitating postpartum depression in this country. What do we do but blame the victim of course: blame it on hormones!

Even if you agree your baby is lucky to be alive, and yes, even if you are thankful for the doctor's skill, and yes, even though you didn't have to go through a painful delivery, you still missed out on the thrill of accomplishment.

It's like a marathon runner who falls and breaks his ankle just as he reaches the finish line... or a mountain climber who falls only minutes away from reaching the summit. You wanted to climb to the mountain peak yourself, not just hear about it.

Having a c/section is like having someone else open your Christmas gifts...

> "Hey, guess what was in your parcel under the tree? A baby boy. Yeah, no kidding! Hold him? No, you can't hold him yet! Since I was the one who opened the parcel, I know best how to look after it."

You might go through a process of grieving over what you lost when your baby came into the world not unlike the loss we face when someone leaves the world. You must face your pain when someone you cared about dies if you are to get over it and get on with your life. Sometimes it is too painful to face at first, and the grief doesn't hit you until later, after the shock wears off. If you do your best to act strong when people are around, it *is* just an act. People will say, "My, she's taking it well." Nonsense. If you put on an act, denying the pain in your heart, keeping "a stiff upper lip," it takes longer to get over it. Then later, after the funeral, when your friends have had their little cry and gone back to their own lives, you'll be all alone with your grief. The best thing to do is to just face it, dive right in, encounter the pain, take on the grief in its wretched, choking agony, wallowing in the pain. That's what family and friends are for, to support you and hug you while your heart breaks. Oh, how it hurts! It is exhausting, but very cleansing, very healing.

Compare this to your loss in childbirth. You try to ignore it but it just doesn't go away. The emotional pain festers like a boil under the skin. You need to pop the zit—ouch! It hurts more at the time, but goes away faster in the long run.

After you have allowed yourself to wallow in justifiable self-pity for a little while, you feel much better. Of course, wallow too long and you turn into a prune—or drown! You certainly don't want to allow your past to ruin your future, and you can't spend your life whining about your past when your future awaits. So face it, accept it, learn from it, and keep going!

Yours in motherhood,
Sheila

Dear Sheila

Just knowing I'm entitled to feel cheated makes me feel much better. Having "permission" to feel badly about it was a big relief, and I'm ready to move on. In fact, now I feel angry. I am furious at the doctor:

"How COULD you?" I want to say to him, "How could you do this to me when I trusted you? Who do you think you are doing those things to my body like you owned it? You treated me like a broken machine. Do you think you are smarter than God?" I want to scream at him, pound him with my fists, and cry.

The anger at least, is more constructive than self-pity. I want to do something; I want to make sure this never happens again. What can I do? Organize a new group to speak out against unnecessary cesareans? Where do I start?

Love, Kay

PS. Didn't your mother ever tell you not to pop your zits?
Mom said squeezing pimples leaves scars!

Dear Kay

Like always, it's after midnight and I'm finally getting the chance to write. Once everyone is finally in bed asleep and the last of the laundry is folded, it's my "spare time." Normal people would use this time for getting a full night's sleep. Sometimes I wake up with the keyboard imprinted on my face.

I'm not surprised you feel anger about your cesarean. I think it's a good thing, because it's constructive, motivating you to take action. If you don't get angry, you just stay sad, weak, and prone to become another victim. I can see you aren't going to let it happen.

If you want to have a VBAC, go back to your doctor and find out why you had the cesarean in the first place. The real reason. Make an appointment just to talk and ask questions. Was there something wrong with your body? With the baby? Were there any other options? What does he think would have happened if you hadn't had the cesarean? How does he feel about VBAC? Does he think you have a good chance of having a VBAC? Under what conditions? Have you told him how upset you were / are about having a cesarean? Does he care? Does he think your feelings matter at all?

The woman trying for a Vaginal Birth After Cesarean carries some extra emotional baggage. Even if a woman has had a medically-managed birth, at least she knows a baby can, with help, get through her birth canal. The VBAC mom worries whether or not she can. Her doctor wonders too, so he allows her what is called "a trial of labour." This trial, unfortunately, operates with the belief that her uterus is guilty until proven innocent. The doctor is the prosecuting attorney and the labouring woman must act as her own lawyer, pleading her case, begging for a lighter sentence. As judge and jury, the doctor has the final say. Sorry, he says, you have not proven yourself able to deliver this child safely. How can we be sure your uterus won't explode, killing your baby? It can't be trusted, and we must protect the innocent. You are therefore and heretofore sentenced to birth by cesarean section, followed by six weeks of doing no hard labour.

If he hesitates at the idea of you having a VBAC, find a new doctor. If he uses words like, "We'll see how it goes when the time comes," then he's just trying to pacify you. If he isn't certain of the safety of VBAC, find a doctor who believes VBAC is safer than repeat cesarean. If he agrees, but only under certain controlled conditions, find a new doctor.

Know how to find a new doctor? Interview them. Yes, YOU interview DOCTORS! Consider this: You are *hiring* him to provide you with a service. If you don't like the way the car runs, you get yourself a new mechanic, right? If you don't like the way your doctor wants to run your childbirth experience, you get a new doctor. This is YOUR special day, so plan it as you would your wedding, taking charge, deciding who you want to attend, and who you will hire to provide the best service. The doctor will probably deliver hundreds of babies; you only have a few chances. Do it YOUR way, not his! Put yourself in the position of an employer, and find the best guy or gal for the job. You'll soon find yourself starting to feel pretty confident and in control when *you're* the boss over your body and your birth.

I left a doctor's office without even seeing him once, over a petty issue. The nurse asked me to get on the scales, and I didn't see why it was necessary.

"It's just procedure," she said, "All our patients have their weight recorded at each visit."

"But I'm not a patient; not yet," I argued. "I'm just here for a consultation. I don't even know if I want him for my doctor." She looked at me kind of funny. "Why wouldn't anyone want him?" was probably what she was thinking.

"Just get on the scales, please. It's not a big deal."

"If it's not a big deal, why does he insist on having my weight recorded before he talks to me?"

I could see she was getting exasperated. Maybe I should get on the scale, I thought, it's just a scale, and the nurse is getting flustered over it. But on the other hand, if this doctor and his nurse are going to make an issue of something as trivial as weighing me for no good reason, what will happen when I go to the hospital to give birth? Will I be up to arguing with them when I am dealing with intense contractions every two minutes? Suppose they consider Internal Electronic Fetal Monitoring and IV no big deal, standard procedure? Am I being petty? Well, petty or not, minor details can have a major effect on the outcome of labour. I politely told the nurse I would not be seeing the doctor, and left.

I felt so good when I left the doctor's office! I was proud of myself because I didn't wimp out and do what they wanted, petty or not. I don't have to put up with their silly arguments, I thought. I can make my own decisions. I'm not going to waste my time when I've left my toddler at home with a baby-sitter for this interview. The nurse may have thought I was making a mountain out of a molehill, but I tell you, the non-interview made me feel much more in control. I didn't succumb to the pressure to conform, but listened to my gut instinct and stuck to my decision. Maybe the doctor was a nice guy after all, and it was just his nurse who was so finicky, but making this simple choice to leave kept me in the driver's seat. Wow, call me assertive!

The new-found assertiveness was a way of regaining control I felt I lost when I had the cesarean. It gave me confidence in myself. I didn't feel like I *deserved* a cesarean. It just didn't seem fair for a healthy, intelligent woman who took classes in natural childbirth should have to have her child surgically removed. Even dumb animals can give birth with no problems.

One more thing... about squeezing those pimples: Yes, Mom told me it would leave a scar, too. She also told me my breasts wouldn't sag if I always wore my bra! Ha!

Sincerely,

Scarface

Third Base

Hitting Below the Belt

CHAPTER 7

The Joy of Our Sex

> Going to a male gynecologist is like going to a mechanic who doesn't own his own car.
>
> -Carrie Snow
>
> (Quoted in the Penguin book of Women's Humour)

It's been said that it takes nine months for man to come out of a woman, and he spends the rest of his adult life chasing women, trying to get back in! Football coaches have been known to forbid the team to have sexual relations before a game, because it was believed their sexual frustration would make them more aggressive.

It's no wonder men have such a strong sex drive, when the male procreative contribution has but one purpose: to plant its seed in fertile ground.

Women, on the other hand, have a multi-faceted contribution to procreation: ovulation, conception, gestation, parturition, and lactation. The survival of our species has depended on all phases of our female sexual functions. *Every one of these aspects of our female function can be — and usually is — controlled by drugs.*

What happens when women are sexually frustrated? I'm not talking about missing out on intercourse before a big game; I'm talking about an entire generation of women who have had their female sexuality medically frustrated. What effect does it have upon our lives as women if we spend our entire adult married lives taking medicines for the disease of being female? Will there be evidence of aggressive behavior in the female, too?

I'd say so. In recent times, the frustration and discontent among women have made them turn their backs on their traditional status as wives, mothers, and homemakers. Men, it appears, get all the perks in life, all the money, all the power, all the satisfaction. Women, the feminists point out, are mistreated, used and abused for men's gratification. Women are not treated equally. "Why would a woman want to be equal to a man, anyway," some say, "Why lower yourself?"

Something has changed in the past few generations. Women appear to have been content in their roles throughout most of history. Certainly there was oppression and domination – just as there still is today. But with all the opportunities available to women today, there doesn't appear to be a huge increase in personal satisfaction, just an increase in our stress levels.

In the animal kingdom we see no discontent as instinct drives them (the poor oppressed females) to fulfill their roles. Are they oppressed? The mother bird works from dawn until dusk feeding her young. Hormones drive the mammalian mother to maintain close contact with her nurslings and protect them.

We humans have been blessed with superior brains enabling us to consciously decide whether or not to rear children, but we often fail to have the same natural instinct to nurture our young. Why?

It is a well-known phenomenon in the animal kingdom if the mammalian mother does not have immediate contact smelling, licking, nuzzling and nursing the newborn she may abandon it. This appears often where animals are raised in captivity, and humans "help" the birth process. Another problem with captive animals occurs when they have never been exposed to normal nurturing behaviour of their species. La Leche League's New Beginnings Magazine related a story in which a gorilla in Toledo Zoo did not seem to know what to do with her new baby born in captivity. To remedy this, the zoo hired a woman to breastfeed her baby in front of the gorilla until the gorilla caught on to the idea.

Problems occur when our superior brains presume we can overlook our animal instinct. It is just as important for the human mother as it for other mammals to touch, smell, hold and breastfeed her baby in the first moments after birth. This human equivalent to licking and nuzzling[i] has a profound effect on nurturing behavior. The human lack of this animal touch is the reason behind our apparent loss of instinctive behaviours.

When doctors began to render women unconscious for the birth of their children, most women welcomed this escape from the pain. But the drugged mother was unable to care for her infant - which is why hospitals needed nurseries in the first place.

A revealing 1976 study compared two groups of mothers immediately after childbirth. One group was allowed extra time to

---

[i] Some women do actually lick and nuzzle their babies, given privacy. (see Kelly Williams story - pg. 185)

hold and cuddle their babies in the first hour after birth, while a control group got the standard treatment – which at the time was merely a brief glimpse of the baby before it was taken to the nursery. The study revealed mothers who were allowed extra contact with their babies spent more time talking to their babies, cuddling them, and maintaining frequent eye contact. These results were still observed in the mothers a full year after the baby's birth! Their babies also cried 550% less than the control group.[17] The mothers in the control group spent over 500% more time changing, bathing, and generally cleaning the baby – though the "unbonded" babies weren't any "dirtier" than bonded babies!

Why were the mothers in the two different groups concerned about opposite ends of the babies? It was as if the thing that came out of her body was dirty. Dirty, like all the other stuff that comes out of our bodies: sweat, urine, vomit, feces, and blood. After the dirty little baby comes out it is always cleaned up before you get to see him or touch him. Milk soon starts to leak from our breasts, but never mind: we can take drugs to dry it up. Other pills control our fertility, preventing our bodies from releasing those nasty little eggs.

Dr. Cynthia Carver, known for her column in *Chatelaine* Magazine, comments,

> Women have been brought up not only to believe that the sex act is a little bit dirty, but that their own sexual organs and sexual functioning are dirty as well.
>
> Few women have seen or been encouraged to look at their own genitals. Menstruation, the evidence of their sexual maturity and capacity for childbearing, is seen as dirty and undesirable and called "the curse," "wearing the rag" or other derogatory terms....
>
> I have a mirror for women to hold when I do an internal exam and Pap smear. When I offer it to them so they can see their cervixes and the inside of their vaginas, at least half of them respond with, "Yuk, no. It's bad enough that all that stuff's there; I certainly don't want to see it."
>
> ...This shame and disgust so many of us have about our bodies cannot be blamed on the medical profession; it clearly is the product of long conditioning, and has its basis in the male domination of Western Society.[18]

Femininity in Its Fullness

A 1978 La Leche League information sheet reprinted from the *Journal of Tropical Pediatrics and Environmental Child Health* notes the effect of a masculine view of a feminine function:

> It is possibly a touch of male chauvinism that causes professionals such as physicians, psychiatrists, sex therapists, and anthropologists to overlook lactation as an aspect of female sexuality. Sympathy and professional help is available to a woman who has

> difficulty in conceiving or delivering an infant, and to a woman who fails to achieve orgasm in intercourse, yet few therapists ask a woman whether she successfully breast-fed, and no one seems to realize that if she has not, an important aspect of her sexuality has been unfulfilled.
>
> Sexuality for a woman does not only mean sexual intercourse and child-bearing, but it includes lactation because with the delivery of an infant a woman is only just starting on what should be one of the most rewarding, fulfilling and sensually satisfying functions of her sexuality. The erogenous zones of a woman's body are not restricted to the genital area, and she can derive a great deal of pleasure in breast-feeding an infant, particularly one that is more than six months old. Such an infant responds positively to her by patting her body, caressing her face, touching her lips and generally showing its delight not only in the milk she provides but also in the close contact with her.
>
> The pity of it is that we have been given a male's eye view of the process... all the fun, sensuality, and emotional enjoyment has become overshadowed by the technicalities of test-weighing...and how many feeds and at what times."
>
> Women are sensual creatures who have a tremendous capacity for enjoying caresses and skin-to-skin contact with a loved one. Those women who deliberately decide not to breast-feed are denying themselves one of the most sensually satisfying experiences of their lives. Psychiatrists, psychologists, and women themselves could well give thought to the possibility that some of the frustration, discontent, and hostility that many women feel today is not because they are unliberated but because their production of the hormone prolactin has been suppressed and a vital expression of their sexuality has remained unfulfilled.[19]

We know breastfeeding has been totally avoided by at least 20% of all Canadian women and by 6 months postpartum only 20-30% of babies are receiving any breast milk.[20]

Many breastfeeding difficulties originate from the unnecessary rules and restrictions imposed upon the nursing mothers. When breastfeeding is merely an alternative form of nutrition it frustrates both the baby, who can't understand why he is denied the breast; and the mother, who could save time and shattered nerves by silencing much of baby's fussing immediately with her breast. Scheduled, planned meals are fine and even necessary for boot camp and large farming operations, not for new and growing relationships based on love.

Any relationship between two people in which body fluids are exchanged is an intimate, bonding relationship. Sometimes, when a woman feels pleasure so intensely through nursing her baby, she fears such a relationship is incestuous. She's so afraid of what she fears is an unnatural affection, she pushes herself away, coldly only picking up the child for scheduled feedings, or switches to bottle-feeding, where she feels "safe" in her affections toward her child.

One of the tricks La Leche League Leaders use to help mothers who seem to have many problems getting the hang of nursing is to tell them to get naked — at least from the waist up — and get in bed with the naked baby (diapered of course.) For some reason this skin-to-skin contact can help turn things around when the usual information doesn't work. It may be hormones or it may be the primitive feeling of raw nudity helps strip away inhibitions, releasing our stifled natural inclinations. Whatever the reason, it's often just what the anxious mother needs to help her get in touch with her more instinctive self. Another tip is to have a glass of wine or beer, to help her relax so her milk will flow. Notice how these tips are the same ones young lovers indulge in as they get to know each other more intimately?

Breastfeeding is supposed to be pleasurable, and we need to embrace it, not run from it. The Womanly Art of Breastfeeding states,

> "Breastfeeding is the completion of a woman's sexual cycle. There are marked similarities in the way a woman's body responds during breastfeeding and intercourse. It is a fulfilling time in a woman's life.[21]" When the baby suckles, impulses from the nerves travel to the pituitary, the master gland in the brain, by way of the hypothalamus, which is near the pleasure center of the brain. Nature intends for mothers to enjoy breastfeeding their babies.[22]

Having a baby without breastfeeding it would be like having a marriage without sex. I don't deny there are many couples in very loving, devoted, celibate marriages, but I pity them for missing out on a deeper dimension in intimacy which is available to them, if only they would take part.

Let's take a positive look at the joys of our sex which are all too often medically oppressed.

<u>The Joy of Fertility</u>

The birth control pill is a safe and convenient way to control fertility and avoid an unwanted pregnancy. Unfortunately its use has had some unpleasant side effects, and I don't mean just headaches and weight gain. When the Pill effectively removed the possibility of pregnancy, there was little excuse in an amoral society for saving sex until marriage. Sex is used as a recreational indoor sport, or a pastime following dinner dates. They'd be better off playing Scrabble, because the hormones released during lovemaking are designed to create feelings of dependency and attachment, bonding you and your partner emotionally while you bond physically.[23] Recreational sex makes it easier to accidentally fall in love with a very poor partner.

In the animal kingdom males must prove their suitability in strength or a show of feathers before females will allow mating to occur. Humans, however, often rely on unreliable criteria like lust when picking a lifetime partner. Watch an episode of *Jerry Springer* on TV and you'll see an example of the pathetic lows to which desperate women will stoop, fighting tooth and painted nail to keep a man in their bed, no matter how poorly they're treated. Thanks to the Pill, women allow the mating to take place first, followed by the inevitable bonding, and then the brains start working later, all in the wrong order. She doesn't realize until she is miserable in the relationship she made a bad decision based on a good orgasm.

Secondly, there is now no reason or excuse for having several children. More than two or three children are seen as either an unfortunate accident, or poor judgment on the parent's part. People feel quite justified in asking expectant couples with two or more children the extremely tactless question "Was this pregnancy planned?" Or the equally invasive, "You aren't having any more, are you?"[i]

Couples who use natural family planning methods enjoy certain blessings Pill-users can't. They learn to appreciate the body's rhythms and can recognize the woman's signs of fertility. The couple must stay in close personal communication with each other regarding their intimate relations. There is a deeper dimension to lovemaking when the couple knows when they can conceive a baby, and when they cannot.

Many women feel a connection to the moon, the tides, and the earth, because of the ebb and flow, waxing and waning, winters and summers of their cycles. Men are stuck with the ability to father a child every single day of the month, every day of the year! We get a break! We are blessed in the cycle of fertility, because we know there are times we can't conceive.

One woman went to her doctor for frequent visits because of a recurrent vaginal discharge problem. It wasn't until after she learned about her fertility cycles from a natural family planning seminar that she realized her "infection" — which her doctor had *treated* her for! — was really just a normal sign of fertility and ovulation.

A woman who is more aware of her bodily cycles can often tell when she has conceived a baby before she has even missed her period (even though her doctor probably won't believe her).

---

[i] My favourite jaw-dropping answer to this invasive question was to introduce our newest baby as our "middle child."

Women who delay the return of the menses for several months by breastfeeding sometimes are quite happy to resume menstruation after a year or more without it. It's almost a pleasant surprise after having had no cycles for such a long period of time; like being a young girl again. The effect of the monthly cycles are now more obvious to the woman, and she can see clearly how the hormone levels affect her mood, her libido, and her emotions as well as her physical changes.

The Joy of Pregnancy

The notion of pregnancy being an abnormal condition requiring close monitoring and frequent testing is as absurd as saying an erection is an abnormal condition for a penis. It's just part of the wonderful built-in multi-function usefulness of the design!

Since pregnancy is considered a medical condition, we tend to be very clinical about our pregnancies, with little to discuss other than doctors' appointments, measurements, or weight gain. We emphasize the discomforts— swollen ankles, fatigue, nausea, heartburn — and spend little time reflecting on the joys of being pregnant. Complaints are the norm.

But many women feel wonderful during their pregnancies. In spite of the discomforts they delight in their changing bodies! Many enjoy increased libido during pregnancy, whether because of hormones or because of the thrill of a new constantly changing body. Not only is the libido increased, but there are also 40 full weeks — 280 consecutive days — to make love without the nuisance of menstruation or worry of conception! Some women find their hair shinier, their skin glowing, and their energy level increased during pregnancy (as long as you get plenty of rest).

Doctors look at our condition from a medical point of view because of their training. They take little notice of the profound effect it has upon a woman to know there is another human being, separate from her, but growing inside of her body. As a man, can he ever understand the thrill of feeling a life moving inside of you? It starts out like a fluttering of butterfly wings, or like champagne bubbles in the belly. You smile to yourself, thinking, "Hello, baby! I know you're there!" As it grows, you can determine which position the baby is in by the movements and the kicking, the elbow jabs, and even hiccups. You can gently make him move over if you are uncomfortable, the way you might move your sleeping husband if he is taking up too much room in the bed.

The bump in your belly is like a special gift; a surprise you can't wait to unwrap and find out what it is! Take delight in the wonderful changes taking place in your body, marveling at the awesome design. Your breasts swell and your nipples darken as they prepare, all by themselves, for the new baby. You are like a grown, strong tree, full and heavy with ripe fruit, ready for the harvest. Like the farmer who waits for the crop to ripen, you wait patiently for the fullness of time, and then the fruit is perfect: a sweet, plump child with skin as soft as a peach.

The Joy of Birth

Birth is the climax of a woman's sexuality, another womanly fact ignored by the male-dominated medical model of birthing. The idea of birth as being an expression of sexuality may come as a surprise, but it is not new. Sheila Kitzinger has compared childbirth to lovemaking. What doctors call expulsion, she calls climax. We are so conditioned to think of birth as painful, dangerous, and a medical problem to be fixed, it's hard to imagine some women find giving birth pleasurable. Some women have described birth as being like an orgasm, and indeed, some women have actually experienced orgasm at the moment of birth.

Birth, as the climax of a woman's sexuality, is probably the most-drugged aspect of her femininity too. Few women in industrialized societies have experienced childbirth without having their perception of the experience altered by drugs. Women who have an epidural usually describe the sensation of giving birth as "a lot of pressure," and they were relieved they didn't have to feel it. After the birth, they complain of being very tired, and just want to sleep. This doesn't seem to be the case when a woman has an unmedicated birth. Rather than fatigue, which is what you might expect, she is often elated! There seems to be another burst of energy with the birth of the baby.

When we are so frightened of the pain of childbirth, many women choose to avoid the sensations altogether, both the pleasure and the pain. Suppose for a moment what would happen if women were so afraid of having sex for the first time doctors would give epidurals for the wedding night? Or at least a narcotic to make her a little woozy. She wouldn't feel the pain, but neither would she take any pleasure from the experience.

After the honeymoon she could relate how relieved she was to have had the drug, because the intensity of the sensations frightened her. We would all have to have medical supervision during sex to monitor our safety, what with the side effects of the drugs. Older women would sip tea at the wedding shower, nodding in understanding of the bride's fears, and reminding her it really doesn't matter how the semen gets into the vagina dear, as long as it gets there. Some brave souls may indeed endure unmedicated intercourse, but it's not for everyone.

An article in Midwifery Today in 1987 pinpointed this very notion in a parody entitled *Orgasmio*. "If men were conditioned from early childhood that the loss of control with orgasm was disgusting," the article asks, "Would men not be seeking methods of controlling themselves so as not to feel the orgasm?"

Daniel, the man in the story, goes to visit the doctor for assessment on the adequacy of his reproductive organ. The doctor — a woman — treats him with a condescending attitude, causing him to worry and doubt his ability to handle an orgasm. Daniel signs up for classes to help him obtain the goal of "control," where they teach him of the risks and dangers and possible complications involved in orgasm.

> Surely since hospital orgasm had become commonplace (removed from the dreaded contamination of the bedroom), there had scarcely been a death associated with orgasm. It is no wonder so many men died in generations past of penile vesicular attrition, enduring such a complicated process at home...to say nothing of the thousands of sperm who died needlessly when orgasms were unattended by certified personnel. Now, monitored by experts, almost every couple could be assured of a successful orgasm. Why, with all the modern testing, drugs, and surgical techniques, even men with highly inadequate penile dimensions and sperm-count could now successfully achieve orgasm!

When Daniel recognizes the first sign of arousal, he goes to the hospital where his erection is carefully monitored. What happens to him in the hospital is only too typical of what happens every day to women in delivery rooms across the country: embarrassing examinations, invasive tests, warnings and watchful monitoring of every aspect of the event. Finally Daniel's female health-care-provider saves the day when she shows up at the last minute, in time to perform a "glansotomy," a small slit in the end of his penis (equivalent to episiotomy) to prevent the sperm from the damage of "head compression." Daniel and his wife were thrilled with the orgasm and so thankful for the staff help at this dangerous, risky time. They had been so *lucky!*

When I show this story to people I notice very different reactions from men than from women. Women usually laugh and nod their heads, recognizing the absurdity of what we are subjected to in childbirth, while men tend to get upset and even downright angry when they read how horribly the man in the story was treated, and for no good reason.

"Don't you see?" the women cry, "That's what they do to US!"

"Ridiculous!" the men proclaim as they inadvertently cover their genitals, "Nonsense!"

Fulfillment in our sexual roles only occurs when sexuality is totally experienced, recognizing and enjoying the full expression of your female-ness. Equal in the importance of their contribution to the family, but different, the masculine and feminine roles complement each other. We don't need to act like men then try to force men to be more like women, for example by insisting men take equal time in feeding the baby. Feeding is an exclusively female function in all mammals.

Not only can we have great multi-orgasmic sex, but we can also experience the thrill of an awe-inspiring, empowering birth; we can know the joy of nursing a baby, and the cyclic gift of fertility. We women are lucky.

The Madonna - Whore Syndrome

The Madonna-Whore syndrome is a way in which men categorize women into one of two extremes. She is either the Madonna: pure and chaste, wholesome, and a devoted mother; or she is the whore: erotic, sexy, exciting, and sensuous. She can't be both. Some men have sexual difficulties when their wives are pregnant for this reason. He can't picture his sexy wife as a mother, or can't imagine disgracing the wholesome Madonna image with his lust. You can see a touch of this idea on television shows and movies which portray younger women as sexy and the older ones fat and frumpy.

It's even noticeable in the retail stores. It's almost impossible to buy anything designed for pregnancy or breastfeeding other than items manufactured strictly for function — not fashion — and certainly not for sex appeal. Maternity underpants, for example, are just about the ugliest garments you can find in the Sears Catalogue. It's hard to find a nursing bra in anything but the functional, industrial-strength, virginal white brassiere. Most of us have little choice but to spend our entire childbearing years wearing flannel nursing nightgowns imprinted with ducklings and bunnies! This is another unfortunate implication that women cannot be both maternal and sexual, so she ought to return to "normal" as soon as possible. It discourages her from taking pleasure in her normal womanly cycles of childbearing and nursing.

<u>Sheila's Hints</u>: At the lingerie shop in your favourite mall you'll find pretty bikini panties with a v-shaped waistband which fits nicely under even the full-term belly. Then get a silky nightgown with buttons down the front or a low-cut v-neck for easy nursing. Finally, get yourself a pretty, sexy bra made of stretch lace, in sexy black or bright red or any colour you like. They're usually cheaper than nursing bras, too. The lace will stretch out of the way when you pull out your breast for your baby, and you don't have to fiddle with a clasp that takes more hands than you have available. You'll feel prettier all over when you know you're pretty all under.

When it gets to the point it has become overstretched (your bra, not your breast) buy yourself a new one, and hang the expense. Consider the purchase as a "tool." It's a necessary part of your job requirement as a nursing mother. Your husband would think nothing of spending money on a tool that would make his job easier even if he only used it once every few months, but you'll be using yours every day. Besides, a new bra is cheaper than a single case of baby formula.

And when they get completely overstretched — your breasts, not your bra — just tuck them under your waistband and save yourself even more money. Hang the expanse.

CHAPTER 8

There's No Place Like Home

"My sister gave birth in a state-of-the-art delivery room," one man told another. "It was so high-tech that the baby came out cordless."

- Current Comedy (Quoted in Reader's Digest)

Home. The word brings thoughts of comfort, relaxation, familiar surroundings, and people we love. Good food, your own bed, your belongings, and privacy. Escape from the rat race. Security.

The home used to be the centre of life's activities, where the most joyful and sorrowful events happened, surrounded by the closest family members. Sick people were nursed at home, old people died at home, and babies were born at home. Parents worked at the home and children got their education at home.

Things have changed. While home is still a sacred place, we spend more of our lives separated. Parents go to work; children go to school. The youngest go to daycare, the oldest go to nursing homes. Birth and death - the most significant of life's events - occur in hospitals. Most of our lives – from daycare to school to retirement centres - are spent in institutions with our peers. Even schools have exchanged the traditional one-room schoolhouse where all ages learned together and helped each other, to segregating children into large classes with others in their own age group.

Lynn Griesemer comments:

> Being born at home teaches family members the beauty and continuity of life. There is bound to be less fear and mystique about birth when families welcome a newborn immediately into their home

> rather than going to a hospital to give birth. Euphoria, rather than postpartum depression is often reported by couples who have had [home] births.
>
> A family that witnesses the death of an ailing family member in the comfort of their home does not have to deal with unpleasant attitudes from the medical staff of pressure to provide various treatments. The family has the privacy to express emotions and begin the grieving process in a more dignified manner. Those who have experienced birth or death at home have seen how the home offers a better psychological, spiritual, and sometimes physical alternative to an institution[24].

Dr. Mendelsohn, who claims Modern Medicine is actually a type of religion in which we place blind faith, says "If you were set on destroying the family, you couldn't do a better job than Modern Medicine."

> Schools and teachers are sometimes blamed for the destruction of the family, but although teachers and educators are surely part of the army of professionals attacking and crippling our families, the generals are the *doctors*. The doctors are the real leaders because without their sanction, without the blessing of Modern Medicine, none of the family-destroying agencies could *exist*, let alone succeed. Furthermore, Modern Medicine's own Holy War on the family is more devastating and vicious than the schools' ever *could* be[25].

Marian Thompson, founding mother of La Leche League spoke on this at a National Conference in 1976:

> One of the most dismaying things to me about the whole experience was when I went to the hospital, I was so excited. "This is going to be the birthday of my baby!" I kept thinking. I could have been going to have my toenails cut for all they cared. I would have loved one person to say, "Gee… Isn't this wonderful! You're going to have your baby today!" How I would have appreciated just one acknowledgement that this was really a special day for me, just one person who understood and shared my excitement at what was taking place.
>
> I know it's not fashionable to talk about things that can't be measured scientifically, yet many of the advantages of homebirth belong in that category. Unless they've experienced it you can't expect people to understand what it means to give birth to a baby in your own bed, surrounded only by people who love and care about you, and to be in a position to truly celebrate a birth rather than just bravely endure it. The effects of these unmeasurables should not be underestimated.[26]

My First Home Birth Experience

I was surprised when my friend Joanne asked me to attend her home birth.

"Me? You want *me* to come?" I gushed. "I'd be thrilled! I'd be absolutely honoured! Wow! I'd love to! But why me? I've never had a home birth."

"It's attitude, not experience that matters," she answered. "You have the right attitude.

It was late at night, bedtime, when she called to tell me she was in labour. I had to bring my nursing baby along of course, hoping for once in his life he might sleep through the night.

This would be Joanne's third home birth. Her three children were so excited about the birth of their new baby brother or sister they were still up.

Dr. B arrived shortly after I did and found her to be only 5 cm dilated. He suggested breaking her water to speed things up. Joanne said no, she'd just wait. So Dr. B went upstairs to the spare bedroom to get some sleep. I took the children upstairs too, so we could rest until the delivery.

After the children were asleep, I went back downstairs to see how Joanne was doing. She was puttering around the house, finishing laundry — at four o'clock in the morning, and in labour! When a contraction came, she'd call her husband, and he would run over and rub her neck and shoulders, and all she'd do was breathe slow and deep, like she was enjoying a massage. She told me later that with each contraction, instead of feeling fear and wanting to escape the pain, she would say a prayer of thankfulness.

"*Thankful?"* I questioned, "For *pain?"*

"Well, no," she laughed, "Not thankful for pain, but for the contraction. And the stronger the contraction, the better, because each contraction brings my baby closer. I thank God for each contraction, knowing each one brings me closer to holding my baby in my arms." So finally I understood what was meant when I read in childbirth books to "welcome" the contractions.

I watched Joanne with interest as her labour progressed. Her manner got progressively more serious, and she asked me if I could rub her back during contractions. I wasn't rubbing low enough; it was the tailbone needing attention. Rubbing, or just pressing against the tailbone, offers counter-pressure to ease pain as the baby's head presses out the tailbone. It's a sign the baby is moving down.

She seemed lost in concentration. What little was said, was spoken in hushed tones, so we might not interfere with her work of labour. Such a contrast to the images of hospital births with everyone yelling at the mother.

Suddenly, with seriousness in her voice, she said softly, "Get the doctor; I'm pushing."

Up the stairs I ran, two at a time and knocked at the door, calling Dr. B. Joanne followed me, her legs wide apart as she went up the stairs, as if the baby's head was already coming. She really could have stayed downstairs, but had her bedroom prepared for the baby's coming.

Joanne had a birthing stool: a small padded, horseshoe-shaped seat which helps the mother be in sort of a squatting position. She had placed on an armchair to raise it high enough to make the doctor's job easier. An old plastic shower curtain was draped over it, pooling on the floor to protect against wetness. She sat on the stool and supported herself on the arms of the chair so she was upright; more standing than sitting.

"Get me the pan," Dr. B said. I saw the old red dishpan on the floor near the bed, and placed it in front of him.

"The pan!" Dr. B said impatiently, "I need the pan!"

"It's there!" I pointed to the red dishpan.

"No, the PAN!" He motioned with one hand, as if it would help me understand. "The PAN...with the, the 'TOOLS'!"

"It's downstairs on the stove," Joanne explained, amazingly calm, "Just bring the whole pan upstairs." Then she gasped as another contraction hit and called her children to wake up.

Down the stairs I ran, two at a time to fetch the 'tools' which had boiled on the stove to sterilize them. There they stayed with the lid on until needed. Dr. B took a pair of scissors from the pan of now-cool water and used them to break the bag of waters which was bulging outside of her body. Joanne was grunting, pushing, and still calling the children to wake up.

I stepped back to let the children get up close. This would be the third birth her eight-year-old son would witness. I picked up the camera to take pictures as Joanne had asked me to do. The bright flash of the camera intruded on the quiet scene, catching a look of unbelievable serenity on Joanne's face as the round dark head appeared. In the picture, Dr. B is squatting on his heels, his hands cupped to receive the baby. A small bedroom lamp glows behind Joanne's head, outlining her long dark hair, and another lamp shines brightly on the baby's dark emerging head. It's like a portrait of the Madonna and child, the doctor bowed before her in reverence of the gift of life.

A splash of water and the baby was born. The cord was very short, so short Joanne could not even turn the baby face-up to see the sex. I placed some protective padding on the bed so Joanne could sit down. She stepped over, carrying the still-attached baby, and sat upon the bed with baby facedown across her lap. Then Doctor B cut the cord and we saw it was a beautiful girl.

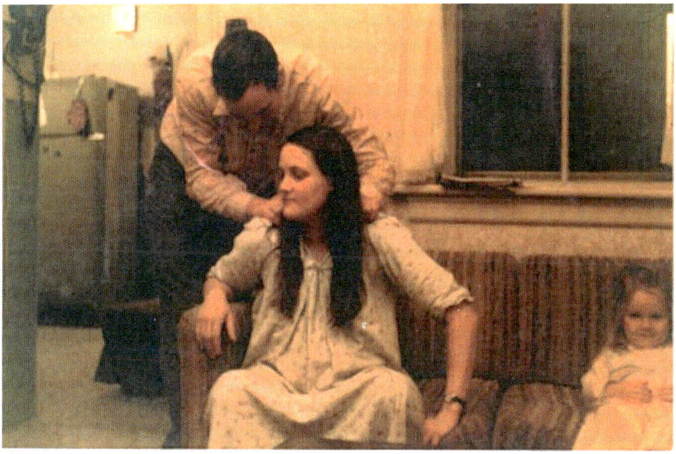

During contractions he would rub her shoulders

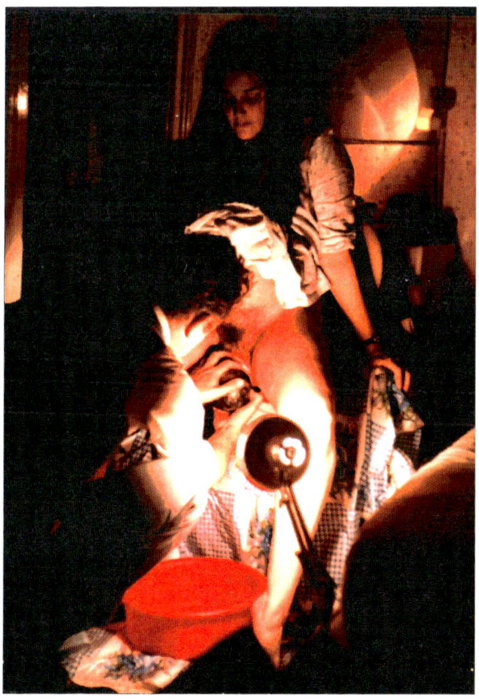

She looked like the Madonna giving birth…

Within an hour, we were all downstairs in the living room again, celebrating with a glass of champagne! Joanne spent the day relaxing on the sofa bed in the living room, like a queen on her throne, her royal subjects bringing her meals. But life went on as usual, the phone ringing with calls about farm business, chores to be done, and some very excited children jumping on the couch, fighting over who gets to hold their new baby sister.

Home Birth - Finally!

I was leaving Radio Shack with my purchase one slushy Saturday in March when another contraction hit. I stood in the doorway letting a cold blast of air into the store, and smiled to myself, realizing I was in labour for sure. I finished running my errands quickly so I could get home, and make sure I took a nap, remembering how tired I had been 2 ½ years earlier during the last labour. Contractions woke me up every 15 minutes for the next couple of hours, but I got up to make supper feeling quite refreshed.

Bert was planning on going to a hockey game, so the boys and I went along to the arena too, since labour was mild and I figured the baby probably wouldn't be born until the next day. I wanted to keep track of my contractions so I borrowed the Fisher-Price watch with a timer Joshua got for his fifth birthday a few weeks earlier.

Contractions started coming every five minutes at the game. By the third period they were getting pretty strong and I was finding it hard to sit still on the bleachers, and squirming and fidgeting in my seat. Bert kept glancing over at me to see how I was doing.

"What's the matter?" his friend asked.

"Oh, nothing," Bert replied nonchalantly, "She's just in labour."

Everyone within earshot suddenly jerked his or her heads around to find the pregnant woman. I gave a quick Queen Elizabeth wave of acknowledgement. When the next contraction hit it was quite obvious to all who were watching, as I wriggled and squirmed on the cold wooden bleachers, wanting – *needing* - to get up and walk, but trying not to draw attention to myself. I watched with amusement as people leaned and whispered to each other about the woman in labour in the third row. Men, women and children turned around to look at me, and soon my status seemed to have become of more interest than the playoff game. When the contraction hit and I started to squirm, with all those eyes on me I thought it was quite hilarious and started to giggle. The contractions started to get stronger, and I giggled even more. The stronger they were, the funnier it was. The more I laughed, the stronger they got!

When the game was over, the men quickly disappeared but several concerned women hovered around me. Some wanted to get me out of there and take me to the hospital immediately, leaving Bert to come later. People get so nervous around a pregnant woman! I didn't dare tell anyone I was not going to the hospital. I did not want to face any negative comments, warnings, or horror stories at that point!

Once we got home, it wasn't so funny any more. There must be safety in numbers as they say, because now Bert was alone with me, he was nervous, wringing his hands and fretting. I called the midwife and the doctor to let them know I was in labour. Just then Joanne, my friend whose homebirth I had attended, came over for a visit. She had already had three babies at home, and Bert was greatly relieved. He disappeared to watch TV while Joanne and I sat in the kitchen and drank a pot of raspberry-leaf tea and munched on a huge bowl of popcorn.

My mother, who had been making a maternally concerned pest of herself by calling me at least once a day for the past several weeks to make sure I wasn't in labour yet, called to let me know there was a bad snowstorm blowing outside. She hoped I didn't go into labour because of the storm. I told her labour had indeed started, but I assured her it would still be several hours before anything happened.

I had to get up on my feet during contractions, and lean my hands on the counter. I was doing a pelvic-rocking labour-dance as I had last time. Joanne insisted I get my birth supplies ready and my bed changed in preparation for the birth. I figured it would be a long time yet, fully expecting I would labour all night like last time and have the baby in the morning. She put the two boys to bed for me, in my waterbed so I could use their firmer bed for the birth. We got the supplies ready in the boy's room, laughing about the wallpaper mural of the space shuttle that made it look like I was giving birth in an airport.

The midwife made it through the storm, arriving about 9:30 at night, and the doctor a half-hour later. I put on my "lucky" nightgown, the one I had worn during the last birth. Joanne had to leave to get back to her family, but I had arranged for my friend Terry to come over to help at the birth. She arrived as Joanne left.

I was getting pretty darn uncomfortable and miserable at this point. I got on my hands and knees on the kitchen floor, and between pains squatted on the bottom step of the stairs leading to the bedroom. I told the doctor I wanted to have the baby in the kitchen, right there on the floor, dammit! (I get a little cranky in labour!) Besides, I had just washed the floor that morning.

"I don't care where you give birth," the doctor shrugged, "It's your house." He told me he had just delivered a baby on the staircase the previous week. The mom was comfortable there, holding on to the railing, he said, and he had found it quite easy to deliver, being a few steps below her.

Elana wasn't hobbled by a cast and crutches this time and was wonderful. She was very involved, staying right beside me, encouraging me, and rubbing my back. She had many helpful suggestions to ease discomfort, such as frequently emptying my bladder. I crawled off the floor to go to the toilet for the umpteenth time, but instead I wrapped my arms around Bert's neck and tried to suspend my weight from him. Watching me do this, the midwife announced, "She's ready to push." In the bedroom Dr. O checked my dilation. Elana was right - I *was* fully dilated! Already? I had no urge to push. Since my water hadn't broken yet, he ruptured the membranes. The amniotic fluid was a dark green — meconium — a possible sign of fetal distress. Dr. O and Elana exchanged a concerned glance, and then commanded, "Push!"

Joanne had lent me her birth stool. I placed it on the bed, climbed on, and started pushing, even though there was no urge to do so. With one arm around Elana's shoulders, the other around Bert's shoulders to steady me, I closed my eyes and made the most incredible, earthy, guttural sounds as I held my breath and pushed down, down, down. In no time at all, I felt burning as the head stretched me until I thought I'd split. Terry snapped pictures, Dr. O put hot compresses on my perineum as the head crowned, and Bert gasped an anxious, "Oh God! ...*Please*!!"

But in a moment I was squealing in the high-pitched voice new moms always use.

"A BABY GIRL! A BABY GIRL! A BABY GIRL!" I screamed as Dr. O placed her, hot and wet, into my arms. (Dr. O always keeps silent while the mother discovers for herself and announces the sex of the baby.)

I held her in my left arm, squealing with delight, tears of joy streaming down my face. Sobbing, ecstatic, I reached up my right arm to Bert, trying to hug him. Bert had his arms raised over his head, like a boxer who just scored a knockout, triumphant. He noticed my hand reaching up to him, grasped it and shook it vigorously in dumbfounded congratulations, and ran off to make phone calls.

It was 11:30 pm, about 12 hours since I suspected I was in labour.

Home Birth Recovery

Elana, being a good midwife, works with a combination of modern knowledge and ancient wisdom. She insisted I stay in my bed for at least an hour before I could get up. I desperately wanted to have a quick shower, for I was sitting naked in a puddle of amniotic fluid, having pulled off my wet nightgown.

She weighed the baby on her scale, which is just like a fish scale from the baby is hung in a cloth sling. Eight pounds, 10 ounces. I nursed her for the first time and Terry snapped pictures.

Elana prepared an herbal bath for me, using a combination of herbs known to promote healing, prevent infection, and soothe sore muscles. These herbs are part of the ancient wisdom of midwives, something I've never heard of in the hospital. After previous births, I wasn't allowed to bathe because of the risk of infection, and the baby was not to be tub-bathed until the cord fell off. I climbed into the smelly green/brown water and Elana put the one-hour-old baby in with me. We watched, fascinated, as the new baby opened her eyes and looked around at her new surroundings, slowly stretching out her arms and legs. I couldn't see what the herbs did for me, since there was no soreness or tears anyway, but the baby's cord dried and fell off within three days.

While I was in the bath, Dr. O filled out all the necessary papers, and Elana and Terry put fresh clean sheets on the bed. I put on my new nightgown; one Terry had made as a gift for me, a warm flannel nursing nightgown with a smaller matching version for the baby. I got back on the bed to relax and nurse the baby again, and we all had a glass of champagne and a piece of Birth Day Cake — Elana, Terry, Dr. O, Bert and myself, and my mother who had arrived by this time. Terry said she was impressed by how quiet the birth was. *Quiet?* What about the guttural, earthy, roar that had resonated through the depths of my soul? Just a little grunting was all, she said.

After they tidied up a bit, everyone went home, leaving us alone with our three-hours-old baby between us. It was after three in the morning before we settled down enough from the excitement to sleep. Only a few hours later I heard a pattering of little feet and Joshua was at the door, rubbing the sleep from his eyes.

"Come and see what I've got," I smiled from the bed. He was so excited to see my little surprise nestled in my arm, he ran for his brother and they climbed in bed with us, marveling at their new baby sister.

Bert's entire hockey team came over to see the new baby in the evening when the midwife was making her first post-partum visit. She pleasantly but firmly told them No, they could *not* stay for a celebratory beer, because new mothers need their rest.

"What if we don't go?" one of the guys challenged her.

"I was a bouncer before I was a midwife," warned the slender Elana. They laughed, and then they left, thankfully. One of the disadvantages of home birth is that people forget to keep visits very short. Nobody would dream of having you serve them tea from your hospital bed—or worse, beer.

Elana told me not to go up and down stairs for a week, which drove me crazy, since we were living in a split-level house at the time. I did find she was right, however, because the more physical activity I did, the heavier the flow.

Lessons from birth #3

- A cheerful mood speeds up labour. Giggling at the arena brought on strong contractions.
- I was more relaxed in my own home. The care providers came to me; I didn't have to go to them. There was no worry about when to go to the hospital, no arrangements to make for a baby-sitter, no stress of leaving my children and not knowing when I'd be back.
- I noticed a shift in authoritative power. It's my home; I'm on my own turf and it's my rightful place to direct and control the decisions made in my own home. Even things like the doctor asking permission to use the washroom serve as a subtle reminder of just who are King and Queen of the castle. People treat you with respect in your own home. In the hospital, you're the outsider; you're the one who isn't allowed into the secret rooms of "staff only".
- In your own home you can give birth wherever you want, and in any position you want. Even on the stairs.
- I was surprised to find the homebirth, overall, *less* exciting than the hospital VBAC. The hospital was like an exciting spur-of-the-moment overnight trip; the homebirth was a personal family event, like a birthday party — which is what it was, actually.
- You must listen to your body. If it feels better to keep changing positions every few minutes, then do so. Moving may be just what *your* body needs to be doing to help move *your* baby down into the birth canal.
- I wonder if everyone is as nasty as me. Apparently I get cranky when I'm in hard labour!
- It still hurt.

My Biggest Baby, My Easiest Birth

There was no other way; it simply had to be my due date. I was far too busy the whole month of September, with plans almost every night of the week. After giving a talk about breastfeeding on the 25th there were no other commitments on my calendar.

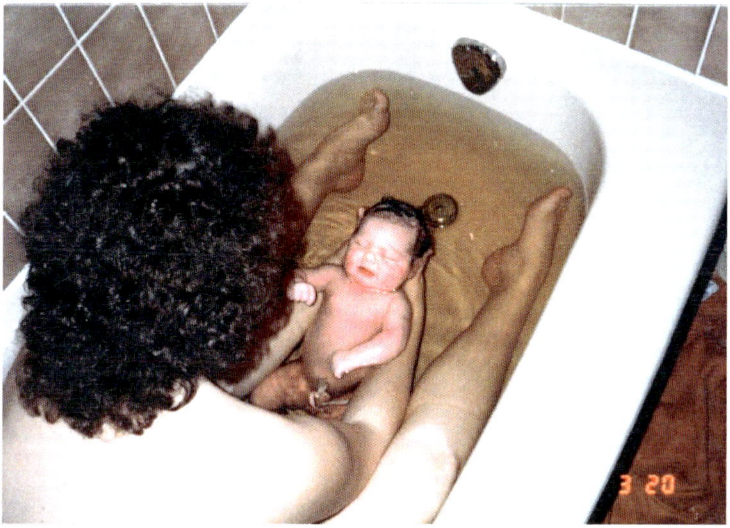

We watched, fascinated as the new baby stretched out her arms and legs in the warm water.

"I feel great this morning," I said to Bert the morning of the 26th as he sipped his coffee, "I even slept really well last night." It was my due date, and the last few weeks had typically been getting increasingly more difficult. I could tell by the weight on my bladder that it was going to be a big baby: my legs ached from the weight of the uterus when I stood, but I couldn't get a deep breath when I sat down.

Not twenty minutes after Bert left for work, I felt a pop and a trickle of warm water down my legs, and then the accompanying shivering and shaking - whether of excitement or a hormonal shift, I don't know.

"Our baby will be born today!" My children begged to be allowed to stay home from school and I agreed to let them if they promised to help me, so they immediately got to work tidying up their toys, sweeping, carrying the laundry baskets and fetching the mail. Meanwhile, I got my supplies ready for the birth and then because I had three pounds of hamburger thawed out in the fridge and knew I'd be heavy in labour about suppertime, I started making meatballs.

Joshua, now age seven, was obviously apprehensive about being alone with his mother about to give birth. Every time I had a contraction, he'd ask nervously, "Are you having the baby right now?"

"No, not for a long time," I told him soothingly, "I'll get really grouchy before the baby comes, because I'll have to concentrate on what I'm doing, and then you'll know it will be soon."

For most of the pregnancy I had been under the care of a GP who happened to live close by. I had hoped he might be interested in attending a home birth, especially since we were neighbours. (Well, in the country "neighbours" means within two miles or so.) But he wanted nothing to do with a home birth and would not support my decision. He tried to convince me how nice and "homey" it would be in the hospital, how things were different now. I went to the maternity ward to see the birthing room for myself. Indeed, it was much nicer than the birthing room I had been in with my first baby, for this one had a wooden rocker, and wallpaper rather than tile walls. The too-narrow bed even matched the rocker. But a flowered bedspread and a wooden headboard didn't fool me. The massive spotlight suspended over the bed, like the ones in the Toronto Skydome, took away from the "homey" atmosphere in my opinion. They might as well have put a lace doily on the fetal monitor.

Nope. Sorry. Once I have given birth at home, and been queen of my own castle, I couldn't go back to their dungeon and be a lowly slave-girl, serving my master by submitting myself to his desires. As his servant girl my job would be the laborious work of pushing a baby out in a difficult, awkward position, so the master could earn his money catching it in comfort.

We'd had an argument over birthing positions, too,[i] so I decided to keep him around as my hired help for stitches and that sort of thing. He's great at emergency medicine, but for a good baby catcher I had to go to the city.

Since moving to our dream home in the country, finances were tight. Our disposable income had gone down considerably and the midwife's fees had gone up considerably. Hospitalization Insurance would pay for a doctor, but we simply didn't have money to spare for a midwife this time, though I would have preferred one.

I was under the care of Dr. B, who had attended Joanne's birth. Good old Dr. Oosterhuis was going to be on vacation, and wouldn't be back until my due date. I had always been overdue, so I didn't mind, but he said no. He said the last month of pregnancy was too important for him to miss, and it would be better to be under one doctor's care. Both Dr. B and Dr. O were trained in the Netherlands,

---

[i] He insisted I would have to be on my back in case he "had to do any pulling." I insisted he wouldn't NEED to do any pulling if he'd get women off their backs!

where homebirth is much more common. (And the rates of infant and maternal mortality are much better than ours are, I might add.)

Dr. B came to visit on a Wednesday afternoon just before my due date, to make sure he could find my place easily. He couldn't.

"It took me over an hour to find you," he grumbled. "Your map is wrong."

"It's exactly forty-five minutes from your office," I said, filling the coffeepot, "Maybe you made a wrong turn somewhere. It's not hard to find the place."

"I don't know how I'm going to manage this if it's during office hours," Dr. B complained, "I can't spend all day driving all over the country when I've got patients waiting. And what if you are in labour all day?"

"So I'll have the baby on a Wednesday, when your office closes at noon!" I answered, indignant. "We can't worry about it until the time comes. Something will work out." He sighed and shook his head. I could see he was beginning to regret he had taken me on as a patient.

Two weeks later, Wednesday, September 26, I called him as soon as his office opened. "I *told you* I'd have this baby on a Wednesday!"

I bustled about between the kitchen and laundry room, making sure the laundry was caught up, making meatballs with the defrosted hamburger, figuring I'd never get around to taking care of these things once the baby was born. It wasn't long before I was getting irritated. Those damn meatballs. I didn't feel like making three pounds of damn meatballs. I was in the middle of a strong contraction, doing my labour dance: leaning over the counter, and rocking my pelvis like a belly dancer, when the damn phone rang. Terry had come to help me out, so she answered it, keeping the heel of one hand on my lower back, pressing where it hurt. It was Dr. B calling to find out about my progress. I was surprised to hear Terry describing my contractions, in a slightly concerned voice, as coming every two minutes and lasting over a minute. No wonder I couldn't concentrate on making meatballs! He said he'd finish at noon and be right over.

My mother came over to help too. Terry took the children outside and gave them lunch while Mom looked after rubbing my back. I stayed on my feet and would lean against the counter doing my pelvic-rocking labour-dance during pains. I felt Mom might be anxious, gauging by her rapid back-rubbing and nervous chatter reminding me how important it was to relax. Between contractions I'd yawn and rest my head drowsily on my arms, almost asleep. She's telling *me* to relax? I smiled to myself and asked to her to rub slowly.

I had told Bert to work until noon and come home then. As soon as he was home I wrapped my arms around his neck and hung, aaah, relieving the pressure in my hips.

"Can I get a sandwich?" he grunted, his back straining. I outweighed him by at least 25 pounds.

"No!"

"I'll just grab a sandwich and —"

"NO!"

"But I'll bring it right back here."

"*NO*!" I shouted. Then the contraction ended, I let go of his neck, turned to Josh, and said sweetly, "Mommy's going to have the baby pretty soon!"

The doctor came in at 12:45, checked me, and announced the baby would be here in about 15 minutes. I didn't believe him. So soon?

I got up on my feet again, and grabbed whoever was handy to lean on, and suspended my weight from their shoulders. It happened to be Dr. B and Bert. We chatted between contractions about my previous birth experiences. I reminded him I'd had a cesarean the first time. He wanted to know the reason.

"Physician Distress," I said, my breath coming in heaving gasps.

He laughed. "You're probably right."

My mother noted that with the newspaper spread all over the place on account of my waters leaking, it looked like we were trying to housebreak a puppy. As the baby moved lower it didn't leak as much. (The baby's head acts like a cork to stop the leaking.)

Another strong contraction hit and I felt something move inside me. (Apparently, it was my bowels. "Oops! Watch your step!" said Dr. B.)

With my arms in a stranglehold around Dr. B and Bert's necks I let my weight be supported on their strong shoulders. It helped relieve the awful, full, my-hips-are-about-to-explode feeling. We talked about my vbac with Dr. Oosterhuis, and Dr. B politely corrected my pronunciation of the Dutch name.

"Not 'Ooooster-house'," he said, "Oh – ster - hois."

"Ohhhhhhh – ster - hoyyyyys" I wailed with the contraction.

"Oh - ster - hoy - is"

"Ohhhhh – ster – hosss! OWWW – STER – YOYZ!!" I bellowed the name out, again and again like a foghorn on a stormy night. Each time I wailed out the name, Dr. B would echo in correct inflection and accent, and I'd trumpet it again, louder, longer, howling it like a wolf at the moon.

"I want you to push on the next contraction."

"No!"

I went over to lie on the bed, on my side, and closed my eyes in an attempt to shut out the embarrassing world where people talk of puppies and pregnancy and poop on the paper. Bert was reclined beside me, stroking my face with his nice cool fingers. The next contraction hit me like a runaway train and I squeezed Bert's hands and held my breath till it passed. It was only when I heard my mother giving an explanation to the boys that I realized I had hollered. "It helps Mommy relax," she said soothingly, "It isn't necessarily painful." *It is, too!* I thought.

Panting like a dog, grunting, and moaning with the next few contractions, I reminded myself over and over again: as soon as this child was born, to call immediately and make an appointment to have my tubes tied. It didn't occur to me until later how the pain was much harder to handle when I was lying down.

Without doing any further vaginal checks, the doctor told me on the next contraction to push.

"NO!" I yelled, and put my foot on his head, and pushed.

One push and I felt my insides shift into my pelvis and the baby crowned. I stopped pushing at the sensation, seconds before Dr. B said to stop pushing. Two pushes and I felt a nose being born, and ears, and a chin. Three pushes and the shoulders came, first one then the other. And, just as he had predicted, 15 minutes after his arrival, I gave birth to a fat baby girl, purple and flailing and smelling sweetly of vernix. Ten pounds, three ounces of warm, wet skin, and deep, dark, blue eyes that immediately looked into mine and recognized me.

We had meatballs for supper.

Reactions to Home Birth

After the baby was born, Bert had some errands to run. We had to have the baby's blood tested to see if it was Rh-negative. If not, I'd need a shot of Rhogam within 72 hours. He also needed to register the birth. He called the hospital to find out where he was to take the vial of the baby's blood for testing (which is milked from the cord, by the way, rather than pricking the poor little newborn baby's heel.)

HOSPITAL: Elgin General Hospital, may I help you?

BERT: Hello. Yes, my wife just gave birth here at home, and —

HOSPITAL: Oh, dear! One moment, I'll connect you with the ambulance!

BERT: No, it's — I don't need —

AMBULANCE: 911 Dispatch; What is the nature of your emergency?

BERT: This isn't an emergency, my wife just had a baby at home, and I just need to know what to do with the blood.

AMBULANCE: How bad is the bleeding, sir? Is your wife conscious?
BERT: No, she's fine, everything's OK, I —
AMBULANCE: Where are you located?
BERT: I don't need an ambulance; I need to know where to take this blood sample. Who can tell me where it needs to go?
AMBULANCE: One moment, I'll put you through....
MATERNITY: Hello, maternity...
BERT: Yes, hello, my wife just gave birth at home. What do I do —?
MATERNITY: Oh my goodness! Is the baby breathing?
BERT: Yes, the baby's fine, but I need to know what to do with this blood.
MATERNITY: How badly is your wife bleeding? Is she conscious?
BERT: Yes, she's fine! Everything's FINE! I just need to know what to do about the baby's blood.
MATERNITY: One moment, I'll put you through...
EMERGENCY: Emergency, Mrs. Blank speaking.
BERT: My wife just had a baby at home. I need to know what to do with the blood from the—
EMERGENCY: Is the baby breathing?
BERT: Yes! She's fine! Everyone's fine! I just need to know what to do with the blood!
EMERGENCY: How much blood is there? Is your wife conscious?

After finding his way to the lab, Bert stopped to buy some flowers for me, and a few cigars to give away, then went to register the birth at the township office. The staff were kind of puzzled. The births are all registered at city hall, they said. So he drove back in town to the city hall, where the staff looked kind of puzzled. That's taken care of in the hospital, they said. The baby wasn't born in the hospital, he said. They were kind of puzzled. Then where in the world, *was* she born? Really? Oh my goodness is everything OK? Is the baby all right? How's your wife?

If the baby was born outside of the city, they said, we'd have to register the birth at the Township Office. Back to the Township Office Bert went, and waited while they searched for and dusted off their birth registry books and entered our baby's name, the first one to be born in the Township of Yarmouth since 1939.

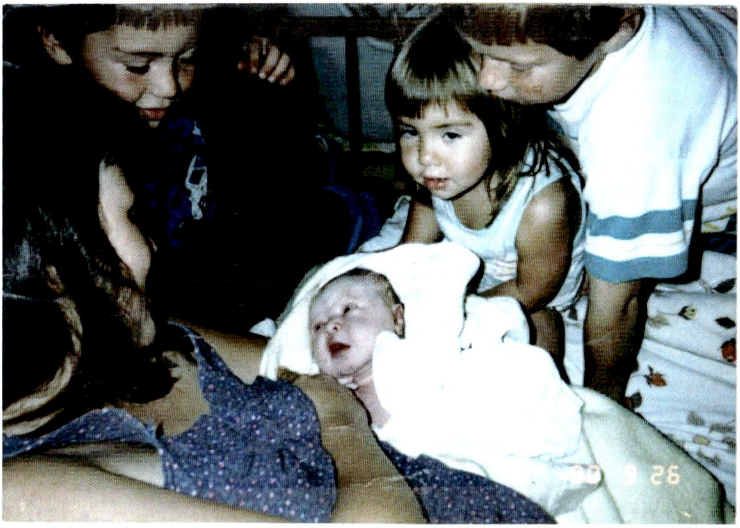

Ten pounds, 3 ounces of warm wet skin, and deep, dark blue eyes that immediately recognized me.

CHAPTER 9

Hospital Birth: Is It *Really* Safer than Home Birth?

Doctors are whippersnappers in ironed white coats
Who spy up your rectums and look down your throats
And press you and poke you with sterilized tools
And stab at solutions that pacify fools.
I used to revere them and do what they said
Till I learned what they learned on was already dead.

- Gilda Radner, Comedian
1946-1989

I am <u>not</u> going to try to convince you to have a home birth. I would never recommend home birth to anyone who is afraid of having a baby at home. The woman who feels safer in the hospital will labour better in the hospital.

That's because fear makes childbirth more difficult. Fear is a fire-breathing dragon that will burn us if we get too close. If the Dragon of Fear is holding you captive, perhaps the truth will set you free. The shocking truth is, the belief that hospital birth is safer than home birth *has never been statistically proven.*

Home births were the norm until the twenties and thirties when the masses began giving birth in hospitals, even though the *mortality rates were — and still are — higher in the hospital* than at home.[27]

As frightened damsels in childbearing distress we cry out to the brave obstetrician to save us from the deadly fire-breathing Dragon of Fear. If we stop running away long enough to face the dragon, once we get a good look at him we might find he is just blowing a lot of hot air.

There are actually three fearsome dragons trying to keep you away from birthing like a queen in your own castle. The first, most frightening dragon is Tragedy, more commonly known as "What If Something Goes Wrong?" Who wouldn't be worried about birth when it can mean life or death? Something Terrible might happen and the baby — or the mother — or both! — could die!

The second dragon is Pain. What if you can't handle the pain? What if you are in horrible pain and can't get pain medication? Why would anyone want to go through such pain anyway, when we have epidurals?

The third dragon lurks in the shadows of the other two and his attack is much more subtle. He is The Unknown. He whispers doubts. "Do you think you have what it takes? Could you manage a medical procedure outside the walls of a hospital? How will you do everything without the medical staff and facilities? Will everything be all right? What will it be like?"

We have enough to do in labour without having to fight dragons. Get ready to slaughter those dragons right now! Don't let them anywhere near your delivery, for the dragon makes labour *drag on.* Clothe yourself in your leather Warrior Babe outfit and take up your sword of courage, and together we'll face those nasty dragons which are trying to keep us from the secret treasure of natural birth.

Tragedy:
"What if Something Goes Wrong?"

This is the most common question about having a home birth. My best answer to the question is with another question: "What if *what* goes wrong?" It's amazing how many people cannot answer that question! Many people don't even know what could go wrong, but are certain it is "something terrible." We are under the impression there is something mysterious about childbirth most of us aren't able to understand, something only the doctor knows. Some unknown terrible thing could happen with no warning and you had better be in the hospital where the doctors and nurses have the equipment and skill to save you and your baby's life. We are afraid of the Unknown! (There's the third Dragon breathing down your neck!)

Franklin D. Roosevelt said, "The only thing we have to fear is fear itself." When a person is afraid, the body becomes tense in a fight-or-flight response: When there's a dragon at the door, you either have to fight it, or flee.

The effect of fear on the labouring woman was discussed extensively in Dr. Grantly Dick-Read's classic book *Childbirth Without Fear*. When a labouring woman is afraid, it causes her muscles to tense. The uterus is a muscle — a huge muscle at delivery. The uterus is trying to do its work, but tension in the woman causes it to work against the tension, causing pain. The excessive pain frightens the woman, which in turn causes more tension, causing more pain.

Dick-Read helped break the fear-tension-pain cycle with education.[28] Understanding what was actually happening in the body made it easier for the women to cope with the discomfort of contractions. Many mothers and grandmothers of this generation of birthing women were rendered unconscious for the actual birth, and had no idea what it was the doctor did to get the baby out. These women would understandably be afraid of the Unknown, and would pass their fears on to their daughters. Women today are usually awake and aware of the goings-on in the delivery or birthing room, but are afraid for different reasons.

You've probably heard of women who were forced to stop pushing, not because *she* wasn't "ready" yet, but because the *doctor* wasn't ready yet. I know a woman who not only was yelled at to stop pushing when she couldn't help it; the nurse actually tried to push the baby's head back inside! Would "something terrible" have happened if the baby slipped out of the mother before the doctor slipped into his gown? Is the mere presence of a medical doctor a guarantee the baby will come out safely?

Childbirth education has done much to prepare women for giving birth and eliminating fear of the unknown. However every one of us who has grown up in front of a TV has been taught to be afraid of childbirth. Almost every TV show and movie you've seen with a pregnant woman in it has a predictable delivery scenario. Suddenly, with no warning, the woman grabs her belly and doubles over in pain. Oh my goodness, she's in labour! She can't talk anymore! She struggles to speak while gasping, grunting or moaning. She can't walk! She must be carried, or someone supports her while she drags her feet. There is a mad dash to get her to the hospital, and everyone is in a panic. It's clearly an emergency.

Next they usually show the birth scene, with all the faces appearing very somber behind surgical masks, and the mother is on her back, still gasping, grunting or screaming. And sweaty, like someone had sprayed her with a hose.

Keep in mind most of what we see in the media of course is unrealistic. Real woman come in all sizes and may have scars, wrinkles, moles and bad hair, but TV women have lean, beautiful bodies, perfect skin, thick, glossy hair, and gravity-defying breasts. Childbirth on TV and movies almost always appears to be an emergency, because it's far more interesting to watch than a normal birth which may take several hours.

Magazines and newspapers also feature stories about life-or-death emergency births. This isn't meant to frighten us, it's just meant to grab our interest. Stories of normal deliveries would be boring, reading like common birth announcements.

If a baby is born in a cab or at home by accident it often makes front-page news. The woman's doctor will be asked for comment, and will remind us how lucky they were that "something terrible" didn't happen. Never does the doctor say, "Well of course everything is fine! Why wouldn't it be?" No, the doctor must remind us birth is a very dangerous affair, requiring his assistance and technology. (After all, if it weren't, he'd soon be out of a job, wouldn't he?)

And yet, of these front-page accidental out-of-hospital births, what is the usual outcome? "Mom and baby are both doing fine!" Keep in mind, these are unplanned, accidental occurrences, and the parents are usually terrified. Sometimes the woman's husband phones 911, where the emergency operator dispatches an ambulance, then coaches the frightened father over the phone on how to deliver his child. Is the 911 operator qualified by experience in emergency childbirth? No! The operator reads the instructions from cue cards!

If mother and baby are both doing fine, why did they have to take them to the hospital anyway? Because we believe birth is a medical emergency and those involved must need medical care.

Fears Begun During Pregnancy

Ultrasound is a fairly recent method of putting fear into women early on in their pregnancies. Many women are more concerned about their pregnancies after the ultrasound, which is supposedly done to reassure them. One woman is told she has "too much" amniotic fluid; another doesn't have enough. Someone else has the dates wrong. Many are told the baby is too small for dates, or too big to deliver vaginally.

Sometimes ultrasounds reveal an abnormality, but should this be a reason for every woman to undergo this test? A recent study in Britain revealed only 55 percent of the babies who were born with an abnormality had been detected during the ultrasound tests. Meanwhile, several fetuses which appeared abnormal in the ultrasound turned out to be perfectly normal.[29] I pity the parents of these perfectly normal babies, who spent months worrying about their unborn child. Rather than being reassured, the victim of ultrasound spends the rest of her pregnancy worrying afraid of the outcome, often without justification.

There are also several blood tests your doctor can do to confirm pregnancy, detect various diseases, and cover his behind. Some doctors subject the woman to unnecessary vaginal exams, or use all the available technology with tests like CVS, amniocentesis, non-stress tests.

One woman in her 60's told me she thought it quite ridiculous, the number of doctor visits during pregnancy by today's women.

When she was pregnant, women generally went to the doctor to confirm pregnancy after missing three periods. Then they'd come and see him again in the last trimester. By the time you are expecting your third or fourth baby, you probably won't need any medical tests to confirm your condition. You won't need tests to hunt for venereal diseases you know you don't have, and you don't need a chart to figure out your due date to confirm what you already know.

Besides, as any mother knows, a simple outing like a doctor's appointment can be enough to exhaust even a non-pregnant mom when there are toddlers in tow.

Studies and Statistics

Did you know that when hospital birth was being defended as safer than home births, all out-of-hospital births were used as a comparison? Those figures included precipitous births in taxicabs and newborns found in trashcans in the out-of-hospital birth statistics.[30] Comparing a well-informed, healthy, prepared couple planning a home birth to a fifteen-year-old drug addict who gives birth in a toilet at the mall is not fair!

A well-known study done in California in 1976 by Dr. Lewis Mehl, MD is a far more reliable comparison of home and hospital births. This study involved 1,046 couples, who were matched, couple by couple, for maternal age, number of previous pregnancies, years of education, socioeconomic status, and risk factors such as presentation (vertex, breech, brow, etc.) multiparity (twins, etc.) previous cesarean, pre-existing hypertension, and symptoms of pre-eclampsia.[31]

This study shows how planned home birth compares to hospital birth:

	Hospital	**Home Birth**
1st Stage of Labour	8 hours average	12 hours average
2nd Stage of Labour	42 minutes avg.	72 min. average
3rd Stage of Labour	5 minutes avg.	22 min. average
birth injuries	30	0
elective induction	22	0
Amniotomy	56	6
Episiotomy	87.4%	9.8%
pain medication	75%	5%
Oxytocin - 3rd stage	95%	24%
Forceps	35%	1.6%
oxygen required	8.9%	1.2%
Cesarean required	8.2%	2.7%*

* cesarean performed after transfer to hospital, of course

You will notice all three stages of labour are accomplished in less time in the hospital than at home. Initially, this appears to be a bonus for the hospital birth. However, the shortened labours are due to the use of the interventions mentioned in the rest of the chart: the amniotomy, episiotomy, oxytocin and forceps. Even though those labours took more time at home, the mothers took much less pain medication.

Take note too the cesarean rate in 1976 was only 8.2%. As you are probably aware, it's 30% or more in some hospitals. But even the low rate of C-Sections is *three times higher* for couples who planned to birth in the hospital, than for couples who planned their births at home.

The study also found that in the **hospital** births,

resuscitation was required	3.7 times more than home births
newborn infection occurred	4 times more than home births
meconium aspiration pneumonia	2.5 times more than home births
newborn respiratory distress	17 times more than home births
fetal distress occurred	6 times more than home births
meconium staining occurred	3.5 times more than home births
shoulder dystocia occurred	8 times more than home births
maternal high blood pressure	5 times more than home births
maternal hemorrhage	3 times more than home births
3rd degree tears	5.5 times more than home births
4th degree tears (into the rectum)	14.6 times more than home births

Why would there be more cases of shoulder dystocia in the hospital?

Why would there be a greater risk of maternal hemorrhage where there is more technology ensuring your safety?

Why is there a greater likelihood of 3rd- and 4th-degree tears dependent upon the location where a woman chooses to give birth?

Does this make sense?

Did they all just get "lucky?"

Or, is there something about *being in the hospital* which makes birth riskier?

Things Your Obstetrician Doesn't Want You to Know

Your obstetrician can brag about the improved maternal mortality rates in the past century, crediting medicine with the improvement. What he doesn't want you to know is that most of the maternal deaths in the previous century were from puerperal fever — an illness *caused by the doctors themselves*! This fatal disease was even reported in the 1700's as being "remarkably infectious in the lying-in hospitals, yet it did not occur at home births".[32] The disease was carried on the hands of the doctors who carried infection from dying patient, to autopsy, to surgery, to vaginal examination, without washing their hands. For years, they refused to believe educated, upper class gentlemen could be guilty of carrying infection on their hands.

Once the bacteria problem was discovered doctors worked on improving their aseptic techniques to the point that by the 1940's every normal, healthy woman having a baby was disinfected and purged like a surgical patient. Not only was this uncomfortable, unnerving, and unnecessary; it made matters worse. For example, shaving the pubic hair of labouring women was standard practice for decades as it was said to prevent infection during the birth, but research revealed shaving actually *caused* more infection than it prevented! Your doctor wants you to forget that too. [i]

Even though most doctors still disinfect the woman's perineal area during delivery to avoid contamination, there is now some evidence that it actually may *benefit* the baby's immune system to come in contact with normal vaginal germs and even feces. (It seems God had His reasons for not making babies come out of our belly buttons.)

Your doctor doesn't want you to know how the death rate actually *increased* when births first moved from homes to the hospitals.[33]

Your obstetrician doesn't want you to know it was doctors and their technology that caused blindness in low birth weight babies.[34]

He wants you to forget about the DES they gave to pregnant women and claimed it was a safe drug with no side effects. He hopes you have forgotten about the thalidomide babies born with no legs or no arms because of a drug deemed safe for pregnancy.

Your doctor doesn't want you to worry about how many of the "necessary" interventions of today will be proven wrong tomorrow, or that many of the procedures he uses today are harmful.

Most doctors are nice people who want the best for their patients. Having faith in modern obstetrics they have been taught that without their assistance, women would suffer more.

Here is an example from their obstetrical bible as it appeared in 1976:

---

[i] I was shocked to find out via the internet some hospitals *still* routinely shave and give enemas to their labouring women! I thought these ridiculous and humiliating practices went out of fashion the same time as disco dancing.

> This encirclement of the largest diameter of the fetal head by the vulvar ring is known as *crowning*. Unless an episiotomy has already been made, the perineum by now is extremely thin, and almost at the point of rupture with each contraction. .... *Failure to perform an episiotomy by this time only invites perineal lacerations and some degree of permanent relaxation of the pelvic floor with its possible sequelae of cystocele, rectocele, and uterine prolapse*[35]. [Emphasis added]

Since 1976 studies showed routine episiotomy caused more problems than it solved. Take a look at what the updated 1997 version of the same book says:

> "One commonly cited but unproven benefit of routine episiotomy is that it prevents pelvic relaxation, that is, cystocele, rectocele, and urinary incontinence…"

The source of the "commonly cited but unproven" benefit was THEIR OWN TEXTBOOK! Doctors don't even want their own students to know who made this error! And I believe the so-called benefits were *dis*proven, not unproven.

By 1997 at least six studies had proven routine episiotomy is associated with an *increased* incidence of anal sphincter and rectal tears.[36] The rate of episiotomy has decreased – but not enough. Today's lifesaving technique is tomorrow's "unproven benefit." Are you willing to risk a tear into your rectum?

In her keynote address at the First National Husband/Wife Homebirth Conference, Marilyn Moran, author of *Birth and the Dialogue of Love*, and *Pleasurable Husband/Wife Childbirth* reminded the audience:

> "Doctors won't be saying things in two years that they are saying today, because they aren't saying things they said two or three, or ten years ago...
>
> "My first seven births… I was medicated hours ahead of time and didn't wake up until hours later... I knew nothing, saw nothing, felt nothing except the stitches, which I felt for weeks afterward. However…
>
> "Who gets Scopolamine and Demerol and so on, that WE got? It was later found out that these are *not* good substances to get into the bloodstream of the baby...so therefore the doctors CHANGED what they were promoting as Gospel Truth.
>
> "I remember in the nursery...the nurse would squirt some Phisohex on the scalp, rub it in and clean the scalp...and said "Don't be worried if you don't rinse it off, because it's antiseptic." Not many years later, with another baby, the nurse said, "Be SURE you get the Phisohex off...It causes cradle cap." A few years later it was found to cause brain damage.

Your doctor doesn't want you to know there are risks of giving birth in the hospital with him in attendance. A doctor will emphasize the risks of home birth to scare you into having your baby in the hospital. Besides, his obstetrical training teaches him childbirth is dangerous and requires medical assistance. One prominent obstetrician who authored an obstetrical textbook said "I have often wondered whether nature did not deliberately intend women to be used up in the process of reproduction, in a manner analogous to that of the salmon, which dies after spawning."[i]

The Politics of Hospital Birth

There is a common misconception that women stopped giving birth at home because hospital birth was much safer. This is far from the truth, according to the research done by the Ontario Government's Task Force on the Implementation of Midwifery.

> One thing that is clear from many different mortality surveys... is that the progression from the popular birth culture to modern obstetrics took place during a time when, for more than three decades, medical birth in hospital was statistically more dangerous than birth accomplished at home in the traditional manner. The popular notion that midwives yielded to modern obstetrics because it was shown to be safer is therefore in error.[37]

Most of the people currently alive on this earth were born at home. Babies have always been born at home, surviving and thriving long before the medical profession claimed childbirth as a medical event. Sometimes there were tragedies, and sometimes babies died, and sometimes mothers died. Today, with all our new diagnostic tests, technology, and surgical procedures available, sometimes there are still tragedies, and sometimes babies die, and sometimes mothers die. The hospital still cannot guarantee your safety and survival and they cannot prove better outcomes.

Because of consumer demand — meaning women like you and me demanded changes — Health & Welfare Canada set up a task force on the Implementation of Midwifery in 1987. The statistics they gathered in their research showed time and time again, in every report, *every* study of home vs. hospital births both in Canada and other countries, there were always <u>lower mortality rates in home births</u>. The shocking truth is that mortality rates were higher in doctor-attended home births than midwife-attended home births, and <u>highest</u> in hospitals.[38]

Physicians liked to explain the embarrassing statistics away by saying it was because the harder cases ended up in the hospital. But in

---

[i] Dr. Joseph DeLee, in *The Principles and Practice of Obstetrics, 1913*

fact, since doctors were more expensive, only the upper class could afford them. Therefore it was often the poorest women, those with inadequate nutrition and no prenatal care who were having their babies at home with midwives, in unsterile conditions, with poor lighting and no plumbing or other conveniences.

Furthermore, in rural areas the "midwives" were often quite inexperienced, since they would only attend a few births a year. They were simply women who came to help out their neighbours when they were in need, knowing the favour would be returned when their time came.[39] The doctor often resented the midwives who received little or no pay for their services, while cutting into what the doctors perceived to be their business.

Because only the upper class could afford doctors, midwives became associated more and more with the lower class. In addressing the Annual Meeting of the Canadian Medical Association in 1931, Dr. W. Henry expounded on this belief by describing midwives as "untrained, unkempt, gin soaked harridans unfit for the work they were supposed to do, and a menace to the health of any woman whom they might attend."

This arrogant attitude was not only unjustified, it was perhaps a better description of the doctors themselves. The *Canadian Medical Association Journal* only two years prior had reported a disturbing study of almost 38,000 confinements revealing the death rates per 1000 maternity cases:

those delivered by midwives 2.8 per thousand;
those delivered by doctors 6.9 per thousand; and
those delivered in institutions 14.9 per thousand.[40]

Who, then, was more of "a menace to the health of any woman whom they might attend?"

Where settlement was new and spread out, and doctors and midwives were few, most ordinary people seem to have been confident about what to do at birth. One woman who kept a diary from 1828 to 1838 described giving birth with only her husband in attendance. After having used a doctor's services for the first two births, she "seems to have felt no need of one from then on".[41]

Birth at home was a happy time, when neighbours and families would come to help the new mother during the delivery and afterward. Like the cold winter, spring planting, and the busy harvest, birth was a normal event in the life cycles of the typical Canadian family.

In a book written by a Canadian doctor in 1942, we see the nonchalant attitude toward the place of birth:

> In earlier times, and in the country districts today, most confinements take place at home. For this, only a midwife, and perhaps

> a nurse, are necessary, though a doctor may be called in if desired... In the city, many people prefer to go to a hospital or clinic, where skilled assistance is always at hand, and the facilities are better. There is however no necessity for this if the home has the necessary conveniences[42].

Dr. C. Lamont Macmillan, in his *Memoirs of a Canadian Doctor*, wrote about how, when he first began his practice in Nova Scotia in 1928, there was no hospital in the area. Maternity cases were all handled in the home.

> In every little community in rural Cape Breton there was a dedicated body of women known as grannies or midwives... For most births they moved into the household and did the housework, as well as looking after the mother and baby. Sometimes they even helped with barn work. For many years after medical services were available to rural Cape Breton, the doctor was called in only when there were complications. The midwife was called first, and it was she who decided whether it was necessary to call the doctor.

Dr. Lamont delivered more than two thousand babies in country homes, some more than a hundred miles from his office. He admits he sometimes wished there had been a hospital available, especially in difficult cases such as occiput posterior, but each time mother and baby did well, and there were no complications. One time a mother had a gut feeling labour would start soon and asked the doctor to come by. Since she didn't appear to be in labour yet, the doctor went for supper at a neighbour's house. The woman suddenly went into labour and gave birth to a 13-lb. baby before the doctor arrived from less than a kilometer away!

Among the Native culture, knowledge of helpful herbs and remedies was widespread and attitudes toward birth were positive. Birth was a time of joy and celebration when families would help the new mother, pampering her with gifts of food and housework while she adjusted to her new baby.

Birth at home is often handled with traditional herbs and folk remedies handed down from generation to generation. Much of the helpful assistance given to birthing mothers is effective, though scientifically unrecognized.

Science is important to doctors. They belittle old folk remedies for common ailments, and disregard use of non-medical practitioners such as chiropractors and naturopaths, as being unscientific. The practice of medicine, we are reminded, is based on fact and controlled study. And yet their theory about birth in the hospital resulting in healthier outcomes has been scientifically proven to be incorrect!

So why didn't they revert back to the safer home births?

First: convenience. It was far easier for the doctor to have the patient come to him, than for him to have to travel to the patient. He did not have to carry his equipment to the home, and he wouldn't have to sit around and wait for the woman to give birth. The nurses could do it, and summon him in time for the delivery, leaving the doctor free to see other patients.

This brings us to the second reason: money. The doctor could earn more money if his patients came to one central location, where he could manage several patients at once, instead of him having to travel to each individual home.

The third reason has to do with power and control. In the home, the doctor was the visitor, but in the hospital he was in his own domain—his territory. He was in charge, especially since only medical people were allowed in the delivery room. With an almost primitive drive, the obstetrician, "faced with the threat of husband-invasion, defends that territory from his very depths—from his instincts," according to Dr. William Hazlett.[43]

With the doctor in control, the husband barred from the delivery room, and the mother drugged into a stupor, he was free to do more procedures without question. It was "The Age of Obstetrical Experimentation." [44] Intervention, rather than being used for special cases, became routine: use of chloroform, episiotomy and forceps, inductions to prevent babies from becoming too large, high forceps deliveries through a partly-dilated cervix, and trying new, virtually untested drugs.

The doctor's reasoning for these interventions was pure arrogance: blame the woman.

> Leading obstetricians announced that the modern woman needed all their interventions because she was dangerously close to being unfit for childbearing. She was psychologically unable to go through the agonies of labour and physiologically too constricted to allow the baby safe passage.[45]

Nurses, horrified by the practices they observed in the delivery rooms, were not allowed to say anything against the doctor. Speaking out against them would break the "ethics of the profession." One nurse in Eastern Canada was taken to court for breach of privilege after she disclosed how a prominent physician was quite drunk when he came into the maternity unit to deliver a baby.[46] Once more, we wonder who the "gin-soaked harridans" as mentioned earlier *really* were.

Dr. Michele Harrison agrees doctors put the blame on the victim for the problems they themselves cause:

> Yesterday on my rounds I saw a baby with a cut on its face and the mother said, "My uterus was so thinned that when they cut into it for the section the baby's face got cut." The patient is always blamed in medicine. The doctors don't make mistakes. "Your uterus is too thin," not "We cut too deeply." "We had to take the baby," (meaning forceps

or cesarean), instead of, "The medicine we gave you interfered with your ability to give birth"[47]

Dr. Mendelsohn adds:

> The doctor never loses, though he plays both sides against the middle and takes bigger risks than necessary. ...If a mother comes into the hospital with her baby in a breech position and the fetal monitor says the baby is in distress, the doctor loses no time in declaring it a life-and-death situation—which indeed it becomes once he starts to perform a Cesarean-section delivery. ...If mother and child survive, [the doctor] is a hero. If they die, well...it was a life-and-death situation anyway.[48]

More recently, the major change in the birth scenario has been the addition of birthing rooms. Set up because of consumer demand, birthing rooms are designed to give women the comfortable surroundings of home, within the safety of the hospital. This should be the answer to everyone's birthing dilemma. But is it? Dr. Mendelsohn doesn't believe so:

> More than ninety-fine percent of births to healthy women ... can and should be done outside the hospital. Yet doctors still scare young mothers and fathers into the delivery-operating room with horror stories of "complications" which are, in truth, statistical fantasies or complications which result from obstetrical intervention. Now that the scare tactics haven't diminished the home birth movement, we see more and more "birthing rooms" appearing in hospitals.
>
> Don't kid yourself into thinking that birthing rooms made up to look just like a real (motel) bedroom are going to make any difference. Once you allow yourself to be lured onto Modern Medicine's turf, they've got you... birthing rooms are not so isolated from the operating rooms that the brass bed can't be rolled into action before the young mother and father know what's going on. If you're on the doctor's turf, you play by the doctor's rules.[49]
>
> If you need the hospital facilities, you should use them. But if you can have your baby in a birthing room, you can have it in your own bedroom. [50]

The Problem with Hospitals

Many of the "Things That Can Go Wrong," only do so because of unnecessary risks taken in the hospital. These interventions are done, not because they are the best, safest things to do for the sake of you and your baby, but because of business and politics, cost-effectiveness and the threat of malpractice. The doctor's biggest concern about your birth is not that you might not have a pleasant experience. His worry is that you could sue him if your baby isn't perfect, putting him out of business. You, therefore, are the potential enemy so it is in the doctor's best interest to insure he has done everything he could do to achieve a good outcome. In a court of law "everything he could do" generally means making the best use of all the equipment he has available.

But in the comfort and familiarity of your home you wouldn't attempt or even *require* most of these interventions. Home-birthing parents recognize the health of their baby has more to do with how well they care for themselves, taking responsibility for their own health to the best of their ability. This is true prenatal *care*, and has more effect on the health of the baby than the doctor's measurements and meaningless tests recorded at prenatal visits.

Mendelsohn warns us:

> "By treating childbirth as a disease, the obstetrician makes his intervention indispensable. If obstetricians acknowledged the fact that more than ninety-five percent of births proceed entirely without complications, more than ninety-five percent of their services would be recognized as unnecessary.
>
> Babies born in hospitals are six times more likely to suffer distress during labor and delivery, eight times more likely to get caught in the birth canal, four times more likely to need resuscitation, four times more likely to become infected, and thirty times more likely to be permanently injured. Their mothers are three times more likely to hemorrhage.[51]

Let's take a look at an all-too-typical hospital delivery to see how this happens.

First, we'll assume you are coming into the hospital in natural labour. More and more women are being induced as soon as the doctor believes the baby ought to be born. I could write an entire chapter on the risks of induction. The number of induced labors in the US doubled during the 1990's, and by 2002 over 40% of all births in the US were induced.[52] If the induction doesn't work, the doctor has to get more aggressive in his intervention to get labour going. Every intervention carries risks, which can lead to problems and progressively more intervention, and higher rates of cesareans.

Suppose you come into the hospital late one night. Your labour has started but you are not dilating very fast. Your doctor may order something to help you sleep through those early contractions. That sounds OK. But does he ask you if you are willing to take the risk, fully aware of the side effects of the drug he gives you may have an effect on the baby's respiratory system requiring resuscitation?

Many hospitals require use of a fetal monitor for at least 15 minutes. "It helps us check on how the baby is doing," they say. That sounds OK. But did you know that every time a hospital starts using fetal monitors, their cesarean rates go up? Or that in spite of the widespread use of monitors and the increased number of cesareans, there has not been any improvement in mortality and morbidity rates?[53]

The nurses suggest you should stay in bed and get as much rest as possible. That sounds OK. Did they tell you on the other hand, that staying upright and walking would help speed up your labour without drugs? That many women find the freedom of movement and exercise relieves tension, eases fears, and reduces pain?[54]

Some hospitals still routinely put an IV in every labouring woman, "just in case." Well, that sounds OK; after all I always wear my seatbelt in the car just in case I get in an accident. But the seatbelt doesn't inhibit my ability to drive. The IV is akin to wearing scuba gear while I drive, just in case I drive off a bridge.

The presence of the IV is not only physically uncomfortable and limits your ability to move freely, but mentally it gives you the impression that you are in danger and may need an emergency operation. If there is an emergency, they can insert it when needed.

The doctor might want to break your water. He says it will help speed things up. That sounds OK. When he asks your permission – and he had *better* ask your permission before he does anything to your body – does he fully inform you he could be introducing an infection? Does he tell you the cord may prolapse when he ruptures the membranes, making an emergency cesarean necessary? Does he remind you how your contractions will become more intense?

Instead of — or as well as — rupturing your membranes, he might suggest using Pitocin to speed up the progress. Does he warn you how using this synthetic hormone can cause uterine contractions so strong it can cause fetal distress, necessitating a C-Section? Did he mention the risk of uterine rupture is greatly increased in an augmented labour? Does he inform you the drug-enhanced contractions are more painful than natural labour, and will soon have you begging for pain medication?

Finally he offers the pain medicine you now need because of the Pitocin-enhanced contractions. Relief sounds wonderful, but does he warn you that it could adversely affect your baby, possibly causing respiratory difficulties? Does he let you know it can cause your baby to be lethargic and have trouble nursing? Does he tell you these drugs have been known to have an adverse affect on intellectual and motor development of the child?[55]

He might offer you the epidural so you will be numbed from the waist down. Does he warn you that the epidural has been related to an increase in neonatal jaundice? That it could give you a headache or a backache which sometimes lasts for several months? That sometimes the anesthesia accidentally travels up instead of down, causing you to have trouble breathing? Does he tell you an epidural tends to slow labour down even more, demanding an increased use of Pitocin?

Does he warn you that you are more likely to need a forceps delivery now, because you can no longer tell when or how to push?

We will assume you have managed to get through your typical labour and the big moment is finally about to arrive! The nurses get you into position: you lie on the delivery table; legs spread wide open, and a bright spotlight shining on your nether regions so the doctor can manage the delivery. This sounds reasonable because it's the only way we know of giving birth, thanks to the media.

But does the doctor explain how your uterus has to work harder when you lie on your back, increasing the need for forceps deliveries? Does he warn you about the increased likelihood of having your skin tear when you lie on your back because it puts more pressure on the perineal tissues than if you were upright? Does he explain that the weight of the uterus will also press on your major blood vessels, making you lightheaded and reducing the flow of oxygen to the baby, leading to fetal distress?

Dr. Mendelsohn shares a secret about the lithotomy position:

> The supine lithotomy position is the basis for most of the interventions that are routine in modern obstetrical practice. It has effectively deprived women of all control over their childbirth experience. It has also made having babies infinitely more difficult, perilous, and painful, and provided obstetricians with countless seemingly rational reasons to come to the mother's aid.[56]

The only person who should be allowed to decide what position will be best for delivery is the woman in labour. *Nobody* but the mother should choose, because only she will know what feels right for this particular delivery. Every birth is unique: babies are varying sizes and shapes and in different positions. Women's bodies and pelvic structures are individual. Left to follow her own instincts, the woman will be able to determine which position will work best for the delivery.[i]

If you do attempt to deliver on your back in supine lithotomy position, you might have one more unnerving thought. Modern delivery beds often have a feature allowing the lower end of the bed to drop away. This means there is nothing but your doctor's hands between your vagina and the floor. I heard about a baby who slipped from the doctor's hands in a local hospital. The baby landed in the

---

[i] Of four home births I have birthed in four different positions: one semi-squatting on a birthing stool, one lying on my side, one sitting on the floor, and one kneeling.

container meant to catch the fluid and placenta. The nurses affectionately called him the "bucket baby."

At this point in our typical hospital birth, you will be instructed when and how to push. Often the nurses will direct you to take a deep breath, hold it, and push while they count to ten for you. Prolonged breath holding, says Henci Goer in *The Thinking Woman's Guide to a Better Birth*, has been shown to compromise the baby's oxygenation.

"Push with the natural urges, breathing as your body directs you," she recommends.

> Expect to have to fight off the troops on this one. Despite the complete lack of evidence for pushing on command or beginning to push at full dilation without an urge, most hospital staff members are convinced that no baby can be born without such pushing[57].

The next step is the episiotomy.

The episiotomy is done with scissors just before the baby's head comes out. Ouch! Some of the most sensitive tissue in your body is cut to enlarge the vaginal opening, to make more room for the baby to come out faster. Well, that sounds ... Ouch! er ... *sort of* OK? Doctor has told you a nice clean cut is better than a jagged scar. Ask him, *For WHOM*? Perhaps he thinks God goofed up when he made the vagina without a zipper.

Has your doctor ever actually pointed out that the main reason he has you in lithotomy position is so he can do an episiotomy, but the main reason you <u>need</u> the episiotomy is because he has you in this position?!

Your doctor *expects* you to tear, so he'll *cut* you first... which sounds to me like breaking your leg so you don't sprain your ankle! It's like getting dentures to prevent cavities! A cut might "prevent" a tear, but so does a gentle, controlled birth, easing the baby's head out the way you ease a tight turtleneck sweater over your head. Yank the sweater over your head too quickly and it could tear. Cut it first and it *will probably tear even farther.*

Does the doctor tell you the episiotomy is usually done long before you would tear, so you don't even get the chance to see whether or not you actually need it before it's done? <u>Williams Obstetrics</u> teaches "It is common practice to perform episiotomy when the head is visible during a contraction to a diameter of 3 to 4 cm."[58]

Is the doctor not aware how skin tears along the weaker membranes and will knit itself together *better* than his straight cut through muscle and tissue? Why does he not know there are more second- and third-degree tears *with* an episiotomy, than without? It's been in the medical literature for years. Perhaps he should tell you the truth: it hurries the birth up for his convenience. Or maybe, the truth is that he was so well trained in when and how to perform and repair an episiotomy, he doesn't know how to deliver a baby without one.

Does he warn you about the risk of infection in the episiotomy? Does he inform you it will be painful to sit on those stitches for days, at best, weeks sometimes, and some women have painful intercourse for *months* after an episiotomy?

The funny thing is: one of the reasons doctors claim to do the episiotomy is to *prevent* damage to the vagina.

In her book Immaculate Deception, Suzanne Arms says

> "…yet despite doctors' admonitions that tissue stretched to the size of a baby's head can never tighten up to accommodate a mere penis, quite the reverse is true. The very muscles that bring the walls of the vagina close together during lovemaking to "grip" the penis also function after birth to tone up perineal tissues and return the vaginal canal to its former size."

Most of us have the impression hospitals are very clean and sterile. Not true! Remember hospitals are places for very sick people to get treatment. How often do people come into your home with tetanus, Ebola virus, E. Coli infection, Lyme disease, C.difficle, and SARS? Who in your home might have AIDS, staphylococcus infection or herpes, and use the same sitz bath as you?

In August, 1998 women who had recently given birth at St. Joseph's Health Centre in London, Ontario had to return with their babies for testing after it was discovered one of the neonatal staff members had tuberculosis. I personally know someone who picked up a tuberculosis infection in her episiotomy incision! About 1 in 20 patients contract a nosocomial infection in the hospital.[59]

What? Your doctor didn't tell you any of this? Was he afraid he'd upset you? How can you consider yourself an equal partner in your health care decisions if he treats you like a child by withholding this information rather than upset you? How can you really regard yourself as a well-informed consumer making the best decisions for the health and safety of yourself and your baby, if you are not told of the *risks* of the procedures before you agree to them?

In her book *A Woman in Residence*, Dr Michele Harrison offers us the following analogy comparing a labouring woman to a dancer:

> Imagine dancers on a stage. Once, doing a pirouette, a woman sustained a cervical fracture as a result of a fall; she is now paralyzed. We try to make the stage safer, to have the dancers better prepared. But can a dancer wear a collar around her neck, just in case she falls? The presence of the collar will inhibit her free motion. We cannot say to her, "This will be entirely natural except for the brace on your neck, just in case." It cannot be "as if" it is not there, because we know that creative movement and creative expression cannot exist with those constraints. The dancer cannot "dance" with a brace on. The straps

around her abdomen, the wires coming from her vagina, change her birth.[60]

The Best for Baby?

In spite of the mother's desire for a good birth experience, let's think about the baby. Isn't the hospital the safest place for the newborn in case something goes wrong?

In case *what* goes wrong? Once more we find many of the bad things happening to babies, happen as a result of medical intervention. A lowered heart-rate in the fetus is one unfortunate side-effect of drugs given to the mother. Fetal distress can also result when the mother is immobilized due to the monitor and/or IV. If she moves around and keeps walking, she is free to shift her hips this way and that, not only relieving pain and pressure as needed, but helping the baby settle deep into the pelvis, the way you move the pickle jar this way and that to get the giant Polski Ogorki out of the jar.

What if the baby doesn't breathe? Again, this is less likely when the mother hasn't taken any drugs. Pain-killing drugs can depress the baby's central nervous system. Most babies breathe without any help from the doctor.

What if the cord is around the baby's neck? This actually occurs quite commonly — about a third of the time — and is handled by simply looping the cord over the baby's head. According to Dr. Mendelsohn, it is not inherently dangerous, whether the cord is wrapped around once, twice, or several times.

> "However, it can be a serious complication when it occurs in the hospital where there has been induced labor, profuse analgesia and anesthesia, and other interventions, and the cord has been unduly compressed. It is not a good reason for going to the hospital, but it is a very good reason for having the baby at home."[61]

What about tying the cord? Tying the cord is the simplest thing of all, and common sense would tell you how to look after it. Within a few minutes the cord goes cold and white like those dead bugs you see under a spiderweb, after the spider's sucked all the juice out of them. You tie a string around it so it doesn't leak, and cut it. That's it. No big deal. When you leave the cord alone for a few minutes, instead of rushing to tie it and cut it while it's still pulsating with blood, there isn't the risk of hemorrhage from the cord. Laura Shanley, in her description of unassisted childbirth did not even bother tying the cord, before she cut it.[62]

Needless fuss over the care of the cord is another hospital-induced worry which turns out to be not only unnecessary, but detrimental to the natural course of healing. A recent study done in Kitchener-Waterloo, Ontario, discovered the hospital tradition of putting alcohol on the cord to help it dry up is useless. Alcohol-treated cords fell off in about 10 days, while those cords which were simply left alone dried and fell off in eight days. There was no difference in the infection rate, either.[63] (Hint: a drop of your wonderful, infection-fighting colostrum on the cord stump kills any nasty germs faster than you can say *antibacterial*!)

Hospital procedures require the neonate be examined. The baby is tested, weighed, measured and recorded, injected with Vitamin K and has prophylactic erythromycin or silver nitrate administered.

By the way, did your doctor tell you *why* he puts silver nitrate or erythromycin in your baby's eyes? It's to protect his eyes from infection you were told, right? Did you know the infection is gonorrhea? Your innocent newborn baby's eyes are burning to protect him from a sexually transmitted disease you are presumed to carry.

Speaking of disease, since your doctor will be handling your vagina and your newborn baby did you ask *him* for a blood test to see what diseases *he* might have?

Dr. Mendelsohn commented:

> I am also concerned that the obligatory ritual of placing silver nitrate in the eyes of the newborn — theoretically to guard against gonorrheal infection — may be responsible for the higher incidence of astigmatism and myopia in the United States than in countries that don't perform this ridiculous rite. It's a useless procedure, and there is no scientific basis to believe that it's safe, yet in many states it is required by law. I tell all my students to comply with the law but to do it by squirting the chemical in the general direction of the baby from ten feet away.
>
> [Silver nitrate causes] a chemical conjunctivitis that prevents the newborn baby from seeing. That doesn't bother doctors because they believe that babies can't see for the first couple of days anyway. The reason they believe that is that the newborn babies they observe have all had silver nitrate put into their eyes. I also believed that they couldn't see until my granddaughter was born in my house and didn't receive silver nitrate. She looked at me and I could tell she was seeing me.[64]

At home there is no hurry to do any procedures. At home the baby is welcomed gently into the world with love and awe into the midst of his own family, as it *should* be. He is greeted by those who love him first, the strangers and the procedures come later. We don't need to put any identification tags on home-born babies! We don't have the risk of getting the wrong baby. Nor do we have to worry about strangers dressed as staff members stealing our baby as has happened before in hospitals. The parents, not the staff, decide who sees or touches the baby.

The Nursery

After spending some time with his parents, the baby usually spends some time in the nursery for observation. This is extremely important we're told, because of things that could go wrong with the baby. That sounds OK, but don't believe it. What nurse would watch your baby as closely as you would? As long as you are not drugged senseless, you can do a much better job of observing the baby in your arms than the nurse can from her desk. You can't keep your eyes off him!

Nurseries were a necessity when mothers were drugged unconscious for the delivery and babies were so badly affected by the drugs they were hung by the heels upon delivery and slapped to make them breathe. Now that safer drugs being used and most mothers are awake for delivery, nurseries should no longer be necessary, and ought to be abolished. Some more progressive hospitals have already done this.[65]

Sometimes the reason given for putting the baby in the nursery is so mother can rest. That sounds OK, but what's wrong with learning how to be a mommy right from the moment you become a mommy? The nurses should care for *you*, so you can care for the baby. If the nurses want to be really helpful, they should give the baby back to you and send you home so you can rest in your own bed or on your own couch. Then the nurses could come over and do the vacuuming.

Normal Maternal Behavior vs. Procedure

After the baby has been weighed, measured, treated with an antibiotic, bathed and wrapped, he is returned to the mother. This is OK because after the nurse finishes her tasks you are free to enjoy your baby for the rest of your life!

But what doctors and nurses don't know because it isn't allowed to happen is that healthy babies, *like all mammals*, can make their way to the breast alone and will latch on to the nipple. And they don't know that the smell and the touch of the baby's vernix-covered skin stimulates a hormonal response in the mother, or that the baby's crawling movements gently massage the uterus, helping it expel the placenta[66]. And no-one can measure how these accomplishments from a minutes-old child will affect the way he perceives the world, and how his parents perceive him.

Call it "bonding," or "imprinting behaviour," or whatever you want, mothers and babies need each other. If we separate animals from their mothers at birth, the mothers sometimes reject their young. In spite of our advanced intelligence, we are not entirely above such instinct. Separation during this learning period affects bonding, your satisfaction and confidence, breast-feeding success and ultimately, your relationship with your baby over the long term.

Your baby will try to tell you he needs to nurse, long *before* he gets to the point of crying. Babies are born with the ability to communicate, and an attentive mother can recognize the signals he makes when he wants her. It might be lip-smacking, a grimace, restlessness, sucking at his fist, kicking his legs, or something else unique to your child. But nursery staff can not and need not pay attention to your baby's non-verbal language. They will bring the baby to be fed when he has had to resort to crying. Thus the baby in the nursery learns loud frantic crying brings a quick response. The baby in your room is communicating with you rather than crying, but the baby in the nursery has been conditioned to scream first when he wants something.

Instead of mothering the baby fully by responding to his attempts at communication, institutionalized childbirth required science to set up a time schedule to determine when babies ought to be hungry and feed them accordingly. I've seen dairy farms operated like that, even feeding animals by a computerized mechanism. It may be good for business, but not for family relationships. Mealtimes are always supposed to be bonding times for family. When the baby only comes out of the nursery for feedings, it reduces the mother to nothing more than a milk-producing food source — just like the high-tech dairy farm. The mother is left with the impression her baby doesn't need *her*, just her food.

Good hospitals are those which treat the mother and baby as one unit. They follow the Baby-Friendly Hospital Initiative set up by the World Health Organization and UNICEF to ensure the optimal support for breastfeeding, including unlimited access to breastfeeding through rooming which allows mothers to care for their own babies.

Did I just say *allowing* mothers to look after their own babies? Sometimes we get the impression the baby belongs to them. If this is the case in your area, don't be afraid to politely, but firmly, assert yourself and remind them of your authority by choosing your words carefully. For example, if they tell you the baby needs some glucose-water, redirect the statement: "I see. You are asking *my permission* to give my baby glucose?"

The mother and baby should be considered as one unit. The baby is still physically dependent on her for its survival, only now the nourishment comes from her breast instead her placenta. Mother needs baby just as much as baby needs mother. His sucking helps contract her uterus by pumping oxytocin and prolactin through her system, which also enhances bonding and attachment behaviour. The mother ought to relax and be pampered while she concentrates on feeding and loving the baby — which is virtually the same thing.

A nursery undermines a woman's confidence. With trained experts caring for the babies, it gives the mother the impression she is not qualified. If it takes an entire team of medical personnel to do the job, how can a new mother expect to feel competent to care for her baby by herself? Who is she to make important decisions regarding the baby's care? She decides she had better get a pediatrician to give her advice, and fast.

> The pediatrician serves as the recruiter for the medical profession. He indoctrinates your child from birth into a lifelong dependence on medical intervention. It begins with a succession of needless "well-baby checkups" and immunizations and then moves on to routine annual physical examinations and endless treatment of minor ailments that would cure themselves if they were left alone.[67]

Because of baby's presumed need to be cared for by medical experts, the new mother is left feeling inadequate and unsure of her ability to care for her baby. In fact, she feels she might be better off to leaving him in the proper care of qualified instructors in daycare; and then she'll go to work and everything will be back to what she remembers. At least she is confident she does a good job there, because she gets paid.

To summarize, the nursery strikes the final blow to a woman's confidence. She is already afraid to give birth, and now she is also afraid to look after her baby. The medical profession has now totally undermined a woman's self-confidence. The very essence of her womanhood, her ability to give birth and raise children, causes her fear and doubt.

Whose Baby Is This Anyway?

Nursery nurses are total strangers to whom you entrust your most precious gift in the world! You don't know their personal habits, their diseases, their like or dislike of babies, or their parenting philosophy! They generally ignore babies fussing. Assuming these experts must know best, some continue this at home thinking it must be correct.

Scheduled breast-feedings go against our natural inclinations to care for our babies and can cause a rift between mother's head and her heart. Calculated feedings are also the result of a masculine influence on a feminine behaviour.

La Leche League has been fighting an uphill battle for years, helping women to enjoy breastfeeding by *freeing* them from the rules and regulations which only complicate the process. The American Academy of Pediatrics finally recognized this in 1997 and stated,

> "Newborns should be nursed whenever they show signs of hunger, such as increased alertness or activity, mouthing or rooting. Crying is a late sign of hunger. Newborns should be nursed approximately 8 to 12 times every 24 hours, usually 10 to 15 minutes each breast."

But, as Catherine Young pointed out in *Compleat Mother* Magazine, the AAP forgot to apologize to the millions of mothers who have tried to breastfeed according to the pediatrician's previous recommendations![68] Too many have felt like utter failures when they were unable to maintain their milk supply breastfeeding under the restricted schedule. It works for some women of course, so the rest blamed their own bodies, or themselves, rather than the ridiculous rules imposed upon them.

It's also interesting to note, when you are in the hospital, the baby supposedly needs observation you aren't qualified to give, but the moment he is home, the experts tell us he is to be put in his own room, and left alone to sleep. Even at home, it appears he is better off if he spends as much time as possible *away from you.*

As you admire your newborn, you are setting the foundations of a new love relationship. Like lovers on their honeymoon, you savor those sweet moments together through all of your senses. You discover each other's bodies, responding to each other's touch, gazing into each other's eyes, tasting each other through kisses and breastfeeding. You drink in his fresh new scent, marveling at how he responds to your voice, and you to his.

"What if you can't handle the pain?"

By now you can see the fearsome dragons are brothers: Tragedy, Pain, and The Unknown work together. When you brought the Unknown into the light for a better look, Tragedy wasn't such a threat any more. With them out of the way, Pain is easy to subdue!

Many more Unknown dragons lurk in the hospital: Where will I be when I am in labour? What will they do to me? Will I be allowed to eat or drink if I want? May I use the phone? Who will be there at the birth? How many people? Will the staff be nice?

Even when they give you your own labour room it's not really "yours." Are you allowed to touch the equipment? Can you lock the door for privacy? Just how settled can you get? Should you unpack your suitcase? Are you allowed to go down the hall? Is it OK if you have a shower? Where are the towels? Will the same nurse who admitted you stay with you the whole time or will it be a different set of nurses between now and delivery? Who is the man that keeps popping in? What's behind the door? Where did the doctor go? Where did she say the shower room is? Where's the toilet paper?

None of these questions face the mother in her own home. You still don't know what to expect in labour of course, but you aren't burdened with the added stress of being in an unfamiliar environment.

Did you hear that? It was the sound of the Unknown dragon shriveling. Take a look: it's not a dragon at all, it's a dragonfly! Slap him like a bug if the fears start to buzz around your head and distract you from giving birth with confidence.

Handling Pain

How do you handle the pain of birth at home?

> *A young Karate student asks his teacher, "What should I do if someone pulls a knife on me?"*
>
> *"Expect to get cut." the teacher replies.*
>
> *The student's mother is outraged. "Why would you frighten children by telling them that?" she asks.*
>
> *"It isn't meant to frighten them" the teacher explains, "It is to prepare them for the confrontation. When you fully expect to get cut, you have already progressed beyond the fear of getting cut. Thus you can get down to the business of fighting your enemy, unimpeded by fear."*

Expect it will hurt to give birth. Don't run from it; move beyond it to your goal.

If you really cannot take the pain, you can go to the hospital, but pain is always easier to cope with in your own home. Have you ever had menstrual cramps or a stomachache so bad you have to leave work or school or wherever, and the moment you got home you felt better? Even though you're still ill, and the cramps still hurt, you just feel better to be at home and not in public. You have the comfort of your own surroundings, your privacy, and people who care with you. You don't have to wear the same image you wear in public. That's what it's like when you have a baby at home. You can "let loose." "Loose" equals relaxed and relaxed means easier, less painful labour.

A headache at work can incapacitate you, but at home, when you can lie down quietly in your own bed, you can find ways to feel better without having to take a pill. Pain is also worse when accompanied by fear. The recurring headache you were sure was brain cancer seemed much easier to bear once you realized you just needed glasses. Put on your glasses and see for yourself, the dragons aren't as scary in real life as they are in legend.

In an article in *Child and Family* Magazine, Dr. William Hazlett points out a reason why women began to fear the pain of childbirth:

> According to Judeo-Christian tradition, what Eve was to suffer was supposed to happen to all women thenceforth, but it worked a hardship on those women who did not suffer in childbirth; it exposed them to

> suspicions of either heresy or wantonness. Catching on quickly, women learned how to avoid suspicion by moaning and crying out louder than their less-fortunate sisters did. After the birth it was they who told the tales of horror and gore, of passing through the Valley of the Shadow of Death. Even today, despite the growth in popularity of natural childbirth methods, although she no longer risks burning at the stake, the woman who accomplishes her birth naturally and with relatively little discomfort, risks comment, quite caustic at times...[69]

According to obstetrician Dr. Carolyn Rawlings, when God punished Adam and Eve, it was not so much "pain" Eve was to endure during childbirth, as it was "toil." This punishment is equal to the man's penalty for sin. Just as Adam must face the difficult work of raising vegetables and bringing forth the fruit of the Earth, Eve now had to do difficult work to bring forth and raise the fruit of her body.[70]

In a mood of joyful anticipation over the coming baby, full of confidence in your ability to give birth, in knowledge of the safety of home birth, and in the security of familiar surroundings, labour pain is easily endured. This is not to say you should expect to have totally painless childbirth, though some women do.

Most of the time when you feel like you can't handle the pain it's because you are in transition and only a few contractions away from pushing your baby out. When you reach this point in a home birth, you don't regret being at home without drugs; you regret having had sex nine months ago.

Now we've slain the dragons called Pain, Tragedy and The Unknown, there is nothing to fear.

Except maybe: The Hospital.

Now don't get me wrong, hospitals are great places to go IF YOU'RE SICK! And it's a fine place to go to have a baby, IF YOU ARE SICK. Giving birth is not a disease, and if mom and baby are healthy and no problems are anticipated, CHILDBIRTH IS NOT A SICKNESS!

It's quite silly when you think about it objectively. We women are *designed* for procreation. We go to the hospital for assistance with something we are *designed* to do. Goodness, we don't worry about squirrels and deer and mice dying during parturition, we know it's natural for them to have a litter every so often and they'll be fine.

Do we not worry about those animals because they don't have problems delivering their young, or do they not have problems delivering their young precisely because we aren't around to worry over them?

Notice, too, animals in captivity have more problems reproducing offspring than those in the wild do.

True Emergencies

What can you do if the frightful, horrible unspoken something DOES "go wrong?"

The answer is, "If something goes wrong, we go to the hospital, of course." The following is an oversimplified answer to the question of what to do in emergency situations.

- If your labour seems to be lasting forever and you are becoming exhausted, you can go to the hospital, and thank God you can be given drugs. Drugs carry risks, of course, but you are willing to take those risks under the circumstances, and be thankful for the medical team.
- If your water breaks and you find the umbilical cord has prolapsed into the birth canal, have someone call the hospital and tell them to prepare for an emergency C-Section. You are on your way already, on the back seat of the car with your butt up in the air to protect the cord from getting compressed. This *would not* have been avoided just by being in the hospital. It's also less likely to happen when your water breaks on its own, than when the doctor breaks it with the amnio-hook.[i]
- Some blood is normal in labour, but too much would be worrisome. Go to the hospital. Estimate how much blood you have lost, because they will ask.
- If you have a gut feeling something is just not right, trust your instinct and leave.
- Hemorrhage far less likely at home, mainly because there isn't the rush to hurry the placenta out before its time. Keep nursing the baby; keep massaging the uterus by hand all the way to hospital by car or ambulance. Have someone else call to tell them you are coming and why. Apparently eating a piece of placenta – or even placing a small piece inside your cheek, will stop a hemorrhage within minutes. I know, you're thinking, "yuck!" But it works for cats and dogs and I bet you'd do it if you had to!
- A cord around the baby's neck is not as horrible as we are led to believe. Slip it off. If it can't be slipped off, tie it and cut it and deliver the baby as quickly as possible.
- Stuck shoulders are eight times less likely at home as the Mehl study shows. Usually a change of position will help. Try standing

[i] You don't *have to* have your waters broken, as some women are led to believe. The baby can certainly be born with the membranes intact. It used to be considered lucky, like a special blessing was bestowed upon the child if the baby was born in a "veil," or the "caul," as it was sometimes called.

up, or on hands-and-knees or whatever position *feels* right. If it becomes necessary, a midwife, doctor, husband, or whoever can reach in a finger and pull one shoulder from under the pubic bone, in a corkscrew maneuver. Ouch! If not, call 911; you may need the Jaws of Life.

- Gasp! The seconds are ticking by and the baby isn't breathing immediately. Less common at home where the baby has not had to deal with drugs administered to the mother. (Seventeen times more likely in the hospital!) Do infant CPR as described in any First Aid Book.

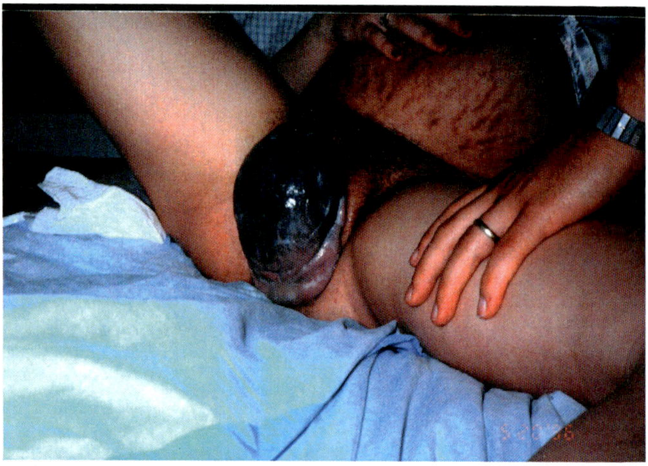

A baby being born with the membranes still intact is rare and used to be considered a sign of good luck.

I was at a home birth where the baby was born white and floppy and not breathing, and those 60 or so seconds were scary. We rubbed the baby's little feet vigorously, rubbed his back, and DID NOT cut the cord, since it's still pulsating blood and oxygen into the baby. The doctor gave him artificial respiration — just one little puff to stimulate him to breathe on his own. I suddenly blurted out a prayer to the Giver of Life, "In the Name of Jesus, baby, BREATHE!" Praise the Lord; he's a great kid, seven years old now and just as perfect as they come. I've often wondered if the baby would have scored better if the doctor hadn't had the poor mother pushing while lying flat on her back like a stranded turtle, knees pulled up to her neck.

This baby, by the way, was an 11 pound home VBAC. The cesarean section was done because she was believed to have a small pelvis, which seemed reasonable: this mother is a tiny spitfire of a woman barely five feet tall. If she can give birth to an eleven pound baby at home, without even so much as one stitch, why are there so many episiotomies for seven-pounders in the hospital?

If You Do End Up In the Hospital

Keep emergency phone numbers handy, clearly visible by the phone. If you have an emergency, have someone call the hospital and tell them you are on your way and why, and they'll be ready. If it's really serious they could call 911 and tell the police so they won't stop you while you speed, or have an ambulance meet you halfway. This would be extremely rare, but it doesn't hurt to have back-up plans.

Most often, if a planned home birth ends up in a hospital, it is a decision made long before any crisis occurs. Sometimes, the hospital staff scolds the parents for the terrible risk they took in planning a home birth. This is nonsense, because the parents did the right and responsible thing, recognizing when medical assistance is required and seeking it. Doctors do their best work in a crisis situation.

Depending on the circumstances, some parents just avoid telling the staff they were planning to have the baby at home, to avoid any confrontation. How are they to know if you've been in labour for 12 hours, or if you progressed very quickly? It happens.

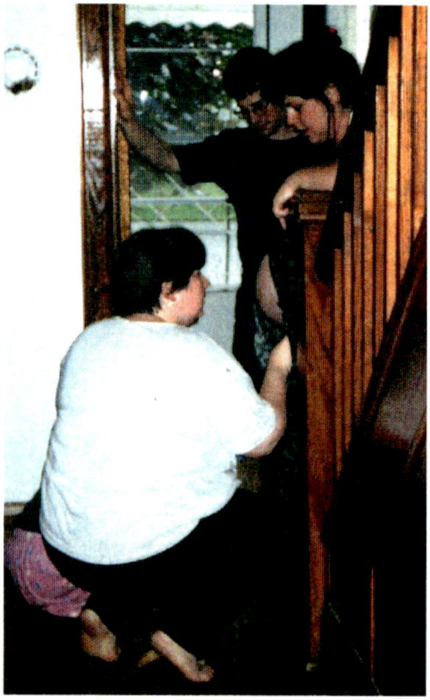

The midwife listens to the baby's heartbeat between contractions.

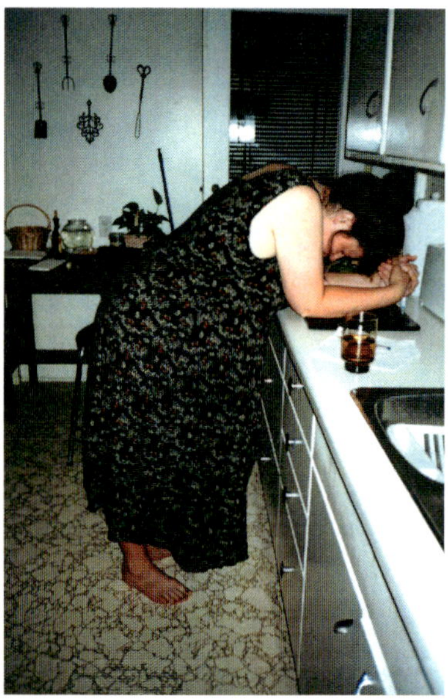

Theresa labours in her kitchen.

CHAPTER 10

The Birth Day Party

When our las' leetle kid she come
(Das numbar 24)
Babette she took ten minutes rest
Den finish scrub da floor

- From a French Canadian Poem

Thus far, I've only talked about the safety of homebirth as if safety is the only reason I would choose it over the hospital. That's like choosing to breastfeed only so my kid will have well-developed dental arches. It's true, but there are many more wonderful reasons making life easier for mom - in both cases!

The Modern McBirth

Hospitals are said to be good places to give birth because of the facilities. Indeed, they are well equipped and have everything a birthing couple might need readily available. But so what?

In the restaurant business, particularly the fast-food business, kitchens are designed specifically for efficient food production in order to serve the most customers with the least effort in the least amount of time. But this doesn't mean we need the same equipment to prepare meals at home!

Admittedly, many of us enjoy the familiar and when we go to these restaurants we know ahead of time exactly what we can expect. We also know what we will get in the hospital, since there's similar standard fare in all franchises. There is some variety to the menu, but you're in trouble if you find yourself in a burger place when you have your heart set on a stir-fry. And what if you really want a candlelight dinner for two on the terrace? Soon they'll install a drive-up birth window where you place your order. "Ok, you ordered the birthing room with a Jacuzzi, and you'll need an enema to go. You want Demerol with that?"

Your house won't have the same set-up as an institution, and it doesn't matter. The home-made, personalized quality and the ambiance are unsurpassed.

Home Birth - Not just safe, but more fun!

At my house, when we plan for the birth, we also plan for the Birth Day Party! Just like any family celebration, we have balloons, gift-wrapped surprises for everyone, cake, and champagne! I have the cake prepared ahead of time, decorated and put in the freezer. The presents are bought and wrapped, waiting for the Birth Day. It's exciting getting ready for the baby and the celebration party when the Big Day finally arrives.

In the hospital, you are in someone else's territory. What is there to do but spend the hours watching the clock, timing contractions, waiting for the second stage of labour? At home, there are things to do, and feathering your own nest for your baby is actually very emotionally fulfilling.

You have little privacy in the hospital. Nurses and doctors can walk in any time. At home, you don't have the unsettling worry of having someone walk in any time. You can sit around in your underwear or stark naked, lie, sit squat, dance, sing off key, or pass gas with gusto.

It's nice to get everything ready so you can relax and just enjoy the baby once it comes, the same way you might get ready ahead of time for Christmas. Depending how you feel of course, whether the labour is hard and fast or slow and steady, you can make sure the laundry is all caught up, the house is tidy, and plan for the next meal. It's exciting to get the baby's tiny clothes and diapers set out, reminding you with each contraction there will soon be a new baby wearing them!

When I was sure I was in labour, I would take the ready-made Birth Day cake out to defrost, and put the champagne on ice. I'd make the bed with clean sheets and place the scissors and shoelace in a pot to boil, to sterilize them for cutting the cord. (Once they have boiled, just leave them in the pot and keep the lid on, and they'll stay clean until you are ready for them.)

If you don't feel up to it, of course, you don't have to do anything. But it is somehow emotionally gratifying to do these things yourself. You can call someone over to be with you to help out, or be alone; it's up to you. You are free to make decisions, to do what *you* feel like doing, and you don't have to ask permission or argue policy with anyone! If you want to make love, it can actually help speed your labour along, as will be explained in a later chapter.

When you birth at home, you don't have a nagging concern about when to go to the hospital. Go too soon, and you'll have a long time to labour there, and a long time to wait. And the longer you are there, the more likely you are to have some interventions. Go too late and you'll have to deal with those horrendous contractions in the car, every little bump in the road magnified so the ride seems like torture. You'll be asked to cooperate with admission procedures, signing papers, undressing, being examined and settled into a room when your contractions are demanding all your attention.

Siblings can be present at the home birth if parents wish

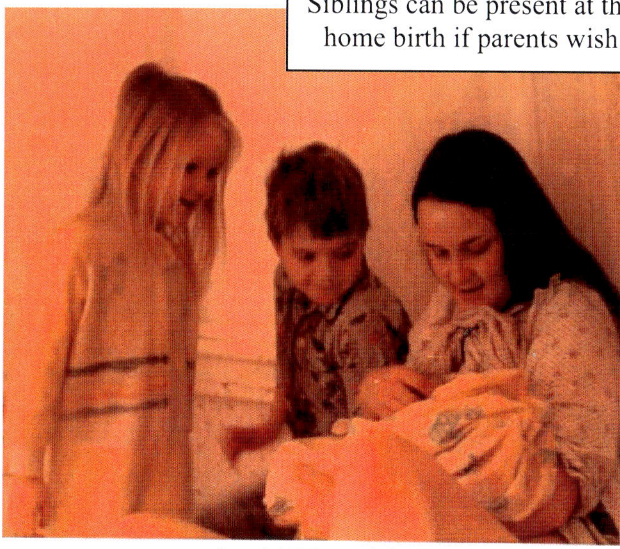

Look! It's a girl!

Birth Attendants

Choose carefully who you want to attend your birth.

Midwives generally work in twos, so there is always one for mom and one for baby. The doctor attending my home birth asked me to have another woman around to help out.

There are several things to consider when you decide whom you would like at the birth.

- Do you want one person, two, or several? Some people enjoy a party atmosphere during labour with close friends to support them and share their special day. Others prefer to keep it as private and intimate as possible.
- What do you want them to do? Housecleaning? Childcare? Backrubs? There's usually a bit of cleanup after the birth: a load

or two of laundry, a few dishes, and making the bed perhaps. Pick someone who won't mind doing a little housework while you and your husband enjoy the baby.

- If you have older children, choose someone who knows your children well and can care for them while you are busy. They might need to reassure your children if you make strange labour-noises, or they just might need someone to get them a drink of juice because "Mommy and Daddy are too busy right now."
- Tell her what you expect from her; let her know of your plans. Pick someone who will honour your wishes. She's there to help YOU.
- In some areas you can hire people who have special training in labour support and post-partum care, known as "Doula's." Or you could just ask your neighbour who had five children of her own.
- Don't make the mistake of inviting someone to your homebirth because it would be a good experience for *her*. This is your day; you have enough to do without performing the perfect birth for someone else's benefit. The attendant is to be there for YOU, not you for her.
- It must be someone who is supportive. If your best friend thinks you are taking a terrible risk, don't invite her. In fact, don't even let her know when you are in labour. You don't want to absorb her worries and fears.
- A friend or neighbour who knows their way around your house and your kitchen could fetch some drinks or snacks without having to ask you questions.
- Have back-up persons A and B and C lined up, in case your first choice of helper is not available, or you need more help than you expected, or in case you have to go to the hospital.
- Who to ask? Find out how your candidate feels about birth. Many think childbirth is "yucky" and want nothing to do with it. Those of us who enjoy pregnancy, babies, and breastfeeding would be thrilled to help you out and consider it a privilege to be invited.

Preparations for the Home Birth

The only thing we had ready for the birth when my fifth baby arrived was a single white shoelace for tying the cord. It cost a dollar at the dollar store.

Something doesn't seem right here: our hospitalization insurance would pay for a hospital, nurses and doctors and dangerous tests like amniocentesis, and all the potentially harmful drugs a labouring mother wants. It will pay for a cesarean, even if it's unnecessary. If the woman wants, insurance will even pay to kill her baby in an abortion. It pays without question for all these procedures, detrimental to both mother and child, but the costs involved in a safe, easy homebirth were my own responsibility. I think somebody owes me a dollar!

The following is a list of helpful items you for homebirth (but as I discovered when caught unprepared, not essential!).

<u>Stuff You Probably Have Already</u>

- Lots of food stored away - so your birth attendant(s) can have something to eat, and so you can peacefully hibernate after the baby is born.
- A firm bed, if the bed is where you want to give birth. A waterbed is too soft. (I spent much of my pregnancy looking for the ideal birthing chair at Goodwill and Garage sales. I wanted something low, so I could be sort of squatting; something with arms so I could raise myself up on my elbows when the baby descends into the pelvis and the hips feel like they might explode; possibly something I could cut open at the bottom. But the baby came early and I had him very easily on the floor.)
- Plastic sheet - or an old shower curtain, or vinyl tablecloth, to protect the mattress (or carpet) from wetness.
- Old sheets and towels - to put over the plastic sheets and absorb fluids. If they're really messy you can throw them out.
- More towels. Or rags. More than you think you'll need.
- Newspapers - also to protect floor if amniotic fluid is leaking. In *Birth and the Dialogue of Love*, author Marilyn Moran describes how to make a pan out of several layers of newspapers by rolling the edges tightly toward the middle. The newspaper pan absorbs fluids and is comfortable to squat on to deliver the placenta.
- Tea Kettle - to "Boil Water!" as they always do mysteriously in the movies.
    1. Make some raspberry-leaf tea. Ancient herbal knowledge shares raspberry-leaf tea is helpful for labour, childbirth, morning sickness, menstrual cramps, and mood swings. Drink daily throughout your pregnancy, and during labour.
    2. Boiling water is also for sterilizing the scissors and shoelace for the cord, and to have warm compresses for the perineum.
- Sharp scissors. The doctor or midwife might have these. I used my hair-cutting scissors.
- A dresser or table cleared off for doctor or midwife use.

- Large bowl or dishpan or other container for the placenta. You can line it with a plastic bag if you like.
- A roll of paper towels - Handy for messes.
- Large garbage bags.
- A shovel. Traditionally, Dad buries the placenta ceremoniously in the backyard, planting a tree over it. We did this, and when we sold our house, we told the new owners about the unique fertilizer we used for the tree. They still call it "The Placenta Tree" to this day.
- Camera, camcorder, or tape recorder for those who want to record the event.
- Heavy-duty industrial strength menstrual pads. You'll need them the first day or so after the birth. When we were caught unprepared, we simply phoned the local "free delivery" pharmacy and had them bring some over. Disposable panties are great too, for the first day or so.
- Thermometer - a good idea to check mom's temp daily - a rise in temperature could indicate an infection.
- A list of emergency phone numbers. Post it by the phone.
- Olive oil - often used for perineal massage. You can put it in a squirt bottle from the dollar store for better aim. Warm it in hot water.
- Soft washcloths or old diapers - for compresses.
- Flashlight - in case of a power failure.

A friend of mine went into labour just after a small tornado had come nearby, knocking the electricity out. They lit all the candles they had, and called a couple of friends to ask if anyone had a nice bright battery-powered light they could use. Before too long, Debbie's house was lit up like a beacon as night grew, the only house in the neighborhood where light poured from its windows out into the yard. The next day, several neighbours came bearing gifts for the new baby and gifts of food for the family. Some of them were people Debbie didn't even know. One lady had tears in her eyes as she told Debbie how touching it was to hear the sounds of a baby being born. Since the electricity was off and the fans and air conditioners not working, everyone had been sitting outside, and neighbours wept as they heard the baby's first cry in the stillness following the storm.

<u>Things You Might Not Have and Might Want to Get</u>

- String or shoelace for tying the cord. I wouldn't pull the 45-inch ones out of your Adidas, but you could sterilize them if you had to! Baby-shoe size is already more than necessary. Shoelaces are soft and pliable like babies, unlike the hard plastic clamps used in maternity wards. Some use embroidery floss.[i]

- Germ-killing soap like Betadine or Phisoderm for hand-washing.
- Infant Ear syringe - to suction mucous.
- Baby Scale - borrow one. Many midwives use a fish scale; it's less traumatic for baby in the sling and they're just as accurate as the cold, hard, flat medical scale babies hate.
- Clothes, washed and clean for the baby. Make sure mom's clothes have easy access for nursing[ii].
- A bottle of champagne for the Birth Day Party.
- A cake; baked and decorated and frozen, ready to thaw while you labour. When we were caught unprepared, my husband ordered a cake and the people at the bakery were so happy for us they gave us the cake for free!
- Gifts for other children, wrapped and ready for the Birth Day Party. Some parents find a video is a good gift at this time, or another toy to keep the children happily occupied, allowing you rest with the baby. Our children insisted the baby got a gift, too. It was usually little socks or booties, so they were satisfied the baby was also enjoying his/her present. Surprise your helper with a gift for her too.

Other Things Some Couples Like to Have

- a large mirror - to watch the birth
- hot water bottle or heating pad
- talc or lotion for back massage
- bendable drinking straws, ice chips to suck
- rocking chair
- Your favorite labouring music.
- disposable diapers
- Vaseline - makes those first black meconium poops easier to clean up. We also used old, worn cloth diapers at first, not only because they are soft, but also because we threw them out rather than try to clean off the meconium.

I have another sneaky suggestion for Vaseline. Spread it on the outside knob of your bedroom door so nobody can barge in uninvited.

Other preparations

---

[i] At one birth I attended, the father braided the embroidery floss using certain colours that had some meaningful significance to them.

[ii] LLL meetings will show you the secrets of discreet nursing - which have nothing to do with hiding anything under a blanket!

- Be prepared to meet with negative reactions. Not everyone will think it is wonderful you just gave birth at home; after all, everyone is sure "something terrible" happens to babies who aren't born in hospitals. The day after baby #4 baby was born we had a plumber over to fix something. He noticed the baby looked very "new" and asked how long we'd been home from the hospital. When I told him we didn't go to the hospital, and the baby had been born at home, he looked very concerned, came close to her and examined her intently for several seconds. "Well," he said cautiously, "She *looks* all right."
- Be prepared to prove the baby is legally yours! We didn't have an official document from a hospital and the lady at the insurance office wasn't sure what to do. To avoid the hassle next time we took a picture of me nursing the baby moments after birth, using a camera that imprints the date. I handed the photo to the lady at the insurance office, along with the doctors' documents, a family photo, and anything else I could think of to prove a live birth, including carrying my baby in a sling to the office.

"Whoa!" she exclaimed at the picture of the new baby all blood-streaked and vernix-covered, and quickly processed the baby's card.

- Be prepared to be firm with visitors. Too many stay too long. I speak from experience. Forgetting I'd still normally be hospitalized, I made tea and served cookies enjoying the company, only to collapse in tears and exhaustion after they left. Yes, I learned the hard way. Next time, I knew to sit still and asked them to make me a cup of tea before they leave.
- Be prepared to *accept* help when people offer. DO NOT be timid about it. If people truly do want to help you, they will be happy to know exactly what they can do to help, when you say, "How nice of you to offer! There's a load of laundry in the dryer to be folded, and could you sweep the kitchen floor for me please?" And if your visitors aren't truly serious about offering their help, then they'll leave, which is even better.

"What About The Mess?"

One lady I know had quick, easy births but said there's no way she would ever have a home birth because of all the mess it would make. You have to wonder how she ever conceived a child if she's so afraid of her sheets getting wet. She'd had a large episiotomy, not because she needed one, but because her doctor is a staunch believer in large episiotomies. An episiotomy makes a big, bloody mess. A baby doesn't. In fact, my doctor made a point of boasting about how *little* mess there is with a home birth. "Look at this room," he said, motioning with a sweep of his hand, "No mess. It's always like this at home."

The bed will get wet from the amniotic fluid. Big deal, you change the sheets. One of the little jobs to do in early labour, part of the emotionally satisfying "nesting," is to make the bed with clean sheets, *twice*. On top of the clean sheets, you put a plastic sheet, and then *another* set of clean sheets. Then, when they get wet during the birth, you simply strip the top layer off. (Not YOU — you get to be queen for a day, ordering your servants around. Get your helper or husband to strip the bed, or your midwife or your annoying neighbour who wants to help.)

The cleanup shouldn't be a big deal. When our baby was born on the bedroom floor, we simply rolled everything up inside the old vinyl tablecloth we had put down to protect the rug. Wet towels, my blood-stained nightgown which was old and worn anyway, meconium-covered receiving blankets, and even the placenta were all rolled up and stuffed it into a big green garbage bag. By law, the placenta must be buried at least three feet down because it is human tissue. Besides, wouldn't you hate to find a dog had pulled it from the trash and dragged it down the street to chew it on your neighbour's porch? If you're going to dig a hole that deep, you might as well do what many families do and plant a tree over. Then you will always remember the unique fertilizer as both the tree and your baby grow.

If it's winter, wrap the placenta and put in the freezer until the ground thaws. One time we put the afterbirth in a large 5-lb. margarine tub. My husband was going to bury it as soon as he got home from work the next day, so we put it in the fridge to keep it from going skunky. The next day I had a Red Cross Homemaker helping with laundry and meals[i]. She made some toast, and looked in the fridge for some butter, and when I heard her shriek I realized she'd found the margarine tub.

Many women have the baby's grandmother come to help out for a week or longer after the baby's arrival. This is the time for grandma to support and encourage the new mother and help with the housework and children. This allows the new mother to rest, recover, bond with the baby, and get breastfeeding established: "mothering the mother so she can baby the baby" as they told us in La Leche League. One woman unfortunately discovered Grandma was so enthusiastic about helping with the new grandbaby, she took over all the baby

---

[i] At the time, Ontario Hospital Insurance would pay for a homemaker for 4 days, since it was thousands of dollars cheaper than a 4-day hospital stay.

care. This left the exhausted new mom to do the housework and cooking.

Hire a homemaker if you don't have a family member to help for the first few weeks. The homemaker can do housekeeping and cook supper while you relax. She might occupy your children with a storybook while you take a nap. (Hint: Have the homemaker make double batches of every meal, one for tonight and one in the freezer for next week.)

The Herbal Home Birth Bath

The Herbal bath is an example of midwifery wisdom doctors don't know about. In the hospital I was forbidden to have a bath and told to wait until after the bleeding stopped and the baby could not be bathed until the cord fell off. At home the baby and I had an herbal bath within an hour. This is another one of the things a mother can do while in labour, putter around preparing the herbs for the bath. Or have your helper do it, rather than stand around and watch you breathe heavily.

This recipe makes enough for 3 baths.

Ingredients:

Plan an herb shopping expedition about a month prior to due date. These are common herbs most often found at health food stores. Buy one large handful each (this is not an exact science!) of dried:

-Calendula flowers or petals
- Chamomile (German or Roman)
- Chickweed
- Plantain Leaves

You may also want to add a whole head of fresh garlic and half a cup of sea salt per bath. These are added just before you get in the tub, but can be bought before also (salt prevents the herbal liquid from freezing properly, so don't add it at this stage). The bath mixture will eventually be placed in squares of cheesecloth (3-4 layers, about six inches on each side), tied, and placed in the bath. You can find cheesecloth at the grocery or fabric store.

Mix herbs well and divide the entire mixture into thirds. Bag and place in an airtight container. Label the container and store it in a cool, dry, dark spot until needed.

To Make Up Prior to Birth:

- Place contents of one bag of herbs into a large heatproof container with a lid (a cooking pot or casserole). You can either tie the herbs into cheesecloth before starting, or afterwards pour the herbal infusion through a fine sieve, saving the liquid.
- Add about 1 litre boiling water to the herbs, let steep covered for 20-30 minutes.
- Remove herbs in the cheesecloth, or strain out of the liquid. Let cool to room temperature, then put into a labeled container and freeze.

To Use:

- Place frozen or freshly made herbal liquid under running tap while filling tub with warm water (save cheesecloth bag of herbs for a compress to enhance healing if needed).
- Add sea salt and/or fresh garlic if desired. (Note: The head of fresh garlic should be crushed or chopped, placed in cheesecloth, rinsed under the running faucet into the tub, and then discarded. The idea is to rinse the garlic juices into the tub and not the pieces).
- Swirl water to mix herbal liquid in and help dissolve salt.

Remember:

- Very hot water is not recommended as it may contribute to dizziness.
- The baby can join the mother if the room is warm and draught-free, but women often enjoy a few minutes in the tub by themselves first.
- Keep the baby submerged up to the neck to keep him/her warm. You can cradle the baby's head in your hand and let her/his body stretch and float in the water.
- Have a helper to take and dry the baby.
- Please don't leave a woman alone in the tub for any length of time in the first few hours after giving birth.

Properties:

- Calendula: astringent (draws tissue together), decreases inflammation, promotes wound healing, and reduces risk of infection (anti-microbial).
- Chamomile: analgesic, antiseptic, decreases inflammation, promotes wound healing (Note: Do not use if you have severe ragweed allergies, as it is closely related).
- Chickweed: promotes wound healing, softens and soothes skin (emollient).
- Garlic: antiseptic, promotes wound healing, reduces risk of infection.
- Plantain: promotes wound healing, astringent, softens and soothes skin.
- Sea Salt: traditionally used for healing and relaxation, trace elements in sea salt (as opposed to table salt) are thought to promote healing.

The Top Ten List

The top ten stupidest questions people have asked me about having a home birth. (My apologies to David Letterman)

1. Would they do a cesarean at home?
2. How do you know being born at home won't damage your child?
3. Will you still get your epidural at home?
4. Who makes the baby breathe?
5. Does the midwife bring the delivery table?
6. Isn't home birth considered a form of child abuse?
7. Do you have to have the baby at home because you don't have any insurance coverage?
8. Aren't you afraid of all the germs?
9. With no nursery, who takes care of the baby?
10. Can I come to watch?

Home

Going all the way

CHAPTER 11

The Marilyn Moran Method

> "We were both raised with strong moral virtues and I always felt dirty with a male OB. I could never understand why, if someone had four more years of school than I, they were allowed to monkey with something I had worked 21 years to keep chaste for only my husband."
>
> - Jane Meyer in *Happy Birth Days*

Stages of Intimacy

Dr. James Dobson, President of *Focus on the Family*, described the stages of physical intimacy a couple goes through from the time they first notice each other until they are fully bonded in marriage. [72]

1. Eye to Body - Noticing someone of the opposite sex.
2. Eye to Eye contact
3. Voice to Voice (Talking)
4. Hand to Hand
5. Hand to Shoulder
6. Hand to Waist
7. Face to Face (Kissing: The beginning of Soul-to-Soul Contact)
8. Hand to Body
9. Mouth to Breast
10. Touching Below Waist
11. Intercourse. (Genital to Genital)

The couple gradually increases the level of intimacy as their relationship builds. The last four would be reserved for times of privacy, hopefully and ideally within the bonds of marriage.

It occurs to me that the offspring of the intimate union then moves in the opposite direction. The baby's life starts at the vagina. The infant requires much hand-to-genital touching in the form of diaper changing, and frequent mouth to breast contact through breastfeeding. Gradually the child moves away from the most intimate of contacts until the child matures to seek his/her own mate and start the cycle again.

Then there's the gynecologist.

The gynecologist has the privilege of going directly from a Number Four handshake on the Intimacy Scale to number 10, without even so much as dinner in a romantic restaurant.

Some women don't mind the gynecological exam. I have always dreaded it. It's worse than going to the dentist. Some people get extremely tense and upset when they have a dental appointment, even to the point of needing tranquilizers to help them through the ordeal. Having some stranger's fingers and steel instruments poking around inside the mouth is extremely unnerving. The mouth is only at number seven on the intimacy scale, and the genitals are "all the way" at number eleven. I think we should be offered a good dose of Valium before going to the gynecologist. Or at least a glass of wine.

What man can understand the dreaded Pap test? They don't have to have their genitals handled and examined regularly by a doctor of the opposite sex like women do!

With as much dignity as a turkey about to be stuffed, you wait for the doctor, legs akimbo and feet in the stirrups. You try to keep your knees together in a vain attempt at modesty, the cold air circulating around your warm parts, covered in nothing but a ridiculous oversized paper towel.

The doctor comes in, pushes the sheet out of the way anyway and pries your knees apart like he's opening the hood of a car. He orders you to slide your bottom right down to the end of the table, closer to his *face*! "Now just relax," he says. Relax? Is he kidding? What if I fart? What if there are tiny pieces of toilet paper stuck there? What if there are strips of long hair like rows of corn on the back of my leg where I missed with the razor? You pull the paper sheet over your face and try to think about something—anything—else.

He thrusts in the duck-bill-shaped thing made of cold steel or hard plastic into the soft tissues of the vagina and jacks it open, like a mechanic about to change a tire. He checks all the parts, and inserts his dipstick for a Pap smear.

How can any woman feel at ease with a strange man between her legs where she can't see him? I try to pretend I'm five years old and playing "doctor." But I never get my turn to play. Unable to see the doctor's face, I imagine he is recoiling in horror, repulsed by some imagined deformity. I realize it's absurd, but what one intellectually understands, and how one emotionally reacts to the invasion are not the same. What else is the poor fellow supposed to do anyway; make pleasant conversational comments on my lovely healthy-looking perineum?

No, I'd much rather go to the dentist. If I have to do it for a stranger, I'd sooner open my mouth than my legs.

Childbirth and Intimacy

"Isn't it embarrassing, having a baby?" asked my seven-year-old, looking at my big belly as the baby inside stretched and moved. "Everybody will be able to see your bare bum!"

I remember asking my mother the same question when I was a little girl. Mom had said no, it's not really embarrassing. When the time comes, she said, you'll be so busy having the baby you won't care — or even notice — who is watching.

Sorry, mom, I disagree.

"Yes, it's VERY embarrassing," I answered, "but you have no choice. You just push hard to hurry and get it over with, and try to forget about the people who are watching." There's no choice in the matter. You have to have someone qualified there to help you give birth. Don't you?

No way, insists Marilyn Moran, author of *Birth and the Dialogue of Love.* She believes the birth of a child, just like the conception of a child, is meant to be a private, loving act between a husband and wife.

Moran believes childbirth is meant to be the completion and fulfillment of the consummation of marriage, the final bonding moment in their union. The man begins the when he plants his seed into her body, but the act is only complete when the woman gives back to the man the fruit from her womb, *in the same manner as the conception.*

How did Moran come to this conclusion? Her first several babies were born in the days when women were heavily medicated to the point of amnesia. Moran was delighted and thought it was a great way to have a baby, even bragging to her friends how she knew nothing, saw nothing, and felt nothing. Then in 1967, when expecting her eighth child, she learned the drugs given to the mother actually had a harmful effect on the baby.

For the sake of her baby Moran took classes to learn about the new "Lamaze" method, and convinced her doctor to allow her to be awake for the birth. Even though her husband was not allowed in the delivery room, she noticed something different in the way she related to her husband throughout this labour. For example, as she was being wheeled to the delivery room, Mrs. Moran grabbed her husband's hand and kissed it. Considering she hadn't kissed his hand but a couple of times in their entire married life, she felt this was a very tender, heartfelt gesture, and a behaviour which had never occurred in previous deliveries when she had been separated from him at the door of the hospital in early labour.

While giving birth, Moran repeatedly twisted and turned her head around, hoping to catch a glimpse of her husband through the window of the delivery room. This was another interesting behavior, she thought. She was surrounded by medical staff tending to her needs. Why was she so desperate for her husband? Wasn't she supposed to be embarrassed to have him see her like this? Was it possible she had a need for him and him alone, a need the nurses and doctors could not fulfill?

It wasn't until three years later that Marilyn's husband was finally allowed in the delivery room. During her labour and delivery she found herself showering her husband with love talk, telling him how wonderful he was, and how happy she was to have him there, even vowing to never raise her voice to him again! The way her own behavior changed in his presence surprised her even more. After all, this was their ninth child together!

Those two unmedicated births were such a revealing discovery of the sensations and emotions of birth, Moran considered perhaps the very act of childbirth is actually a form of deep communication between a woman and her husband. This was "Body language in its most eloquent expression,"[73] an amazing discovery of the sensations and emotions of birth she'd been denied. The drugs had covered so much more than just pain.

Reflecting on these last deliveries she concluded childbirth, while hidden behind the mask of medicine, is actually an intensely sexual experience. The best place for a sexual experience to take place, she decided, is in the privacy of one's bedroom. In 1972 her youngest child was born in there. She was 44 years old at the time.

Her tenth and final birth was so profound in its physical and emotional sensations, Moran was inspired to write a book called *Birth and the Dialogue of Love*, describing the experience of husband-wife homebirth and its effect on marriage.

"Childbirth is not the time for a woman to *get* a baby" says Moran, "but rather the time for her to *give* a baby to her beloved, bringing full circle the action which he had initiated nine months earlier."[74] When the obstetrician steps in between the man and wife to accept this "conjugal love-gift," it leaves a sense of "unfinished business" between the couple, which Moran feels may be an unrecognized source of much of the marital strife couples experience.

But is this marital discord simply due to changes occurring in the sex relationship after childbirth?

Many women confess to having very little sex drive after giving birth. Though the desire may be there, many women report sex just "isn't very good" any more. Usually they complain they are too tired. Lovemaking gets as much enthusiasm as cleaning the toilet; it's just another chore on a checklist of endless, exhausting, repetitive tasks a new mother faces:

- ❑ Nurse the baby
- ❑ Change the diapers
- ❑ Wash the dishes
- ❑ Fold the laundry
- ❑ Bathe the baby
- ❑ Nurse again to put baby to sleep
- ❑ Floss my teeth
- ❑ Have sex to put husband to sleep
- ❑ Try to get some sleep before the baby wakes again

Marilyn Moran's point about shared birth made perfect sense to me. I noticed a change in my husband after the birth of our second child — the first one born vaginally. The cesarean delivery of our first child had physically separated us from each other as well as removing us both from having any active part in the birth of the child we had made together. In celebration of his very first Father's Day I bought my husband a T-shirt on which were emblazoned the words "I'M A DAD!" I was disappointed because he rarely wore it. It wasn't until after the VBAC the "I'M A DAD" T-shirt came out of hiding and he began wearing it with pride. It was his favourite shirt, and he wore it almost every day, even after it was frayed and torn and faded. He didn't give it up until the letters started to fall off and people thought it said, "I A Duh."

It was as if he didn't "feel" like a dad until we had experienced the birth *together*. The surgical birth had reduced us to a position almost like children ourselves, subject to the authority of the medical staff. It was they who took responsibility for the birth. The doctor was the star of a drama in which we were merely players. In contrast, the VBAC was something we had worked at and accomplished *together*, my husband holding me as I pushed, and with both of us being present (and conscious) for the birth.

How Childbirth Affects Marriage

After decades of keeping husbands away from the delivery room, studies were finally done in the 1960's proving the husband's presence at delivery was a crucial factor in making childbirth a psychologically positive time.[75] We should not need to spend several thousand dollars on studies to prove women feel more at ease with their own husband at their private parts, rather than the gloved hands of a strange doctor, intern, midwife, nurse, or OB/GYN.

For several years Marilyn Moran published a newsletter for homebirthing couples. Through the pages of the New Nativity Newsletter, Moran noticed how many of the women who had given accounts of their home births related increased feelings of love and affection toward their spouses. Having found this to be true in her own experience as well, Moran decided to see if there were any measurable difference between the couples who had given birth privately at home, and hospital-birthing couples.

She obtained a copy of the Intimate Relationship Scale; a questionnaire for postpartum couples designed to observe the sexual adjustment following childbirth, developed by Susan H. Fischman CNM and colleagues of the University of Maryland School of Nursing and Medicine. Fischman's results had showed:

> At four months postpartum 84% of the couples surveyed reported having sexual relations "less" or "much less" than before birth.
>
> By one year after the birth, 60% of couples surveyed still reported having intercourse less than before birth.[76]

This was not a surprise, just a statistical documentation of a common problem. "Is There Sex After Children?" is a common theme in parenting magazines. The usual complaint: it's just not very good any more. We're too tired.

Moran sent the same survey to couples who had given birth in their own homes in privacy. The results showed dramatic differences between hospital-birthing couples and those who gave birth in privacy.

Of the home-birthing couples,

> 64% said the frequency of intercourse at four months had not changed at all; and
>
> 21% actually said it was "more" or "much more" sex than before the birth!

By twelve months postpartum,

93% reported having sexual relations *at least as often, or more* than they had before giving birth![77]

Of the mothers who gave birth in the hospital, 55% had reported "fatigue" as the major reason for decreased libido, but only 7% of the homebirth mothers reported the same.

"It's a mystery as to why," comments Marilyn Moran. "Presumably the mothers in both groups had similar demands made upon their time for cooking, cleaning, shopping, and car pooling, in addition to infant care."

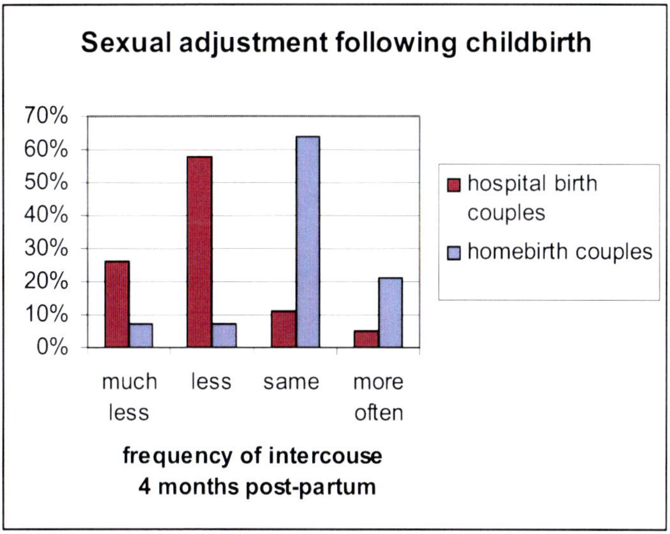

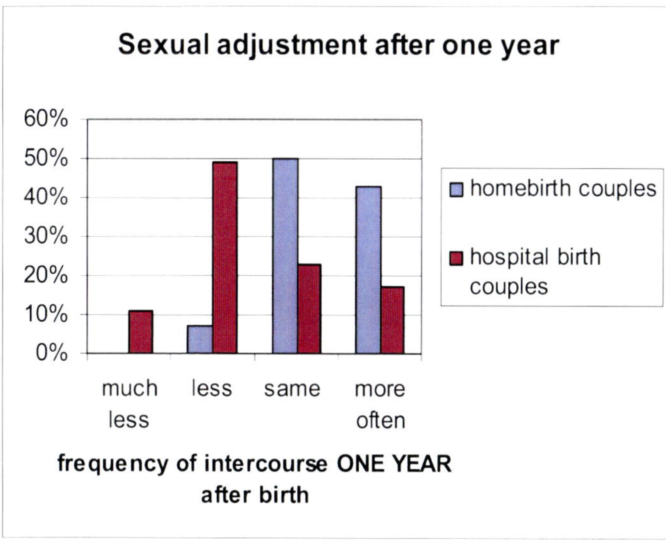

In fact, why weren't the hospital-birthing couples reporting *less* fatigue, since they were the ones who benefited from a few days' rest in the hospital?

Moran blames the medical model of birthing:

> What has robbed sex of its dynamism? It is man's failure to realize that childbirth is as much a part of the marital encounter as is

coitus. Because of his ignorance, man has created a corporeal communication gap which prevents married couples from attaining the level of development that is their due.

A husband ends up cheated and disappointed when his wife hands herself over to the medical specialists. She, too, suffers because of her action. Each and every Adam is entitled to get his rib back. Eve must realize that birth is her opportunity to return Adam's rib. Then no longer beholden to him she will be free to take her rightful place at his side and no separation, no division will exist between them.

Marriage is a pledge of life-long intimacy. When brave, young lovers use the birth experience as a vehicle of a marital intimacy, an exquisite something will be released from the warp and woof of the human fabric and a new world brought into being.

The Need for Privacy

Whether using our genitals for copulation, procreation, or excretion when it comes to private acts most of us want privacy. Patricia Carter forbade even her husband to invade her privacy while she gave birth. In order to give birth easily she said we need to get in touch with our more primitive selves.

Not all of Mrs. Carter's recommendations would be acceptable given today's understanding of prenatal health. She drank alcohol and took sedatives during pregnancy to help her relax. She smoked heavily and barely ate, happily bragging she gained no weight at all during her pregnancy. She even wore a tight corset in hopes of keeping the baby small.

In my experience, mother's weight gain doesn't necessarily change the size of the baby. The pregnancy in which I gained the most weight (50+ lbs.) resulted in my smallest full-term baby; the one in which I only gained 17 pounds resulted in my largest baby at 10 lbs. 3 oz.

Furthermore, a large baby can be delivered as easily as a small one. Just after my fourth (and biggest) baby was born, my family went to the local Harvest Festival to carve pumpkins, decorate scarecrows and sample fresh apple pies. I saw a friend at the Festival and she could hardly believe her eyes when she saw me "out and about" with a four-day-old baby. She had been sore for months after her 4lb. baby was born, from the episiotomy and subsequent tear. She nearly fell over when she found out how big my baby had been at birth – especially when she found out we had ridden our bikes into town!

Carter drank alcohol during labour to help relax both her muscles and her inhibitions. She believed uterine contractions are not supposed to be painful, but only appear so because we expect them to be as a result of our upbringing: we are taught to think sensations in the reproductive organs are "naughty" so we repress them, while pain remains a socially acceptable feeling.

In direct contrast to what the best educated obstetricians would have us believe, Carter's experience indicates the *less* brains one brings to childbirth, the better:

> Even if it hadn't been so trained and educated, the Brain should stay out of this business. What happens to your feet when you watch them dancing? Your fingers when you type? You know how mad and confused it makes you when the boss gives you a job...and then comes and stands over you.
>
> I do not mean here that you strive for disassociation, or to go into some ... state where the brain is cut off from everyday consciousness. Indeed never have you been, or will be, more alert. More aware in all your senses...
>
> I repeat - the Happy Birth is the brainless birth. Is this so strange? Think. Have not your most *brainless* moments been your happiest, your most remembered, the ones in which you lived to the fullest?[78]
>
> The easy birth will not depend upon our strength, our will power, or our brain power. *It will depend upon their absence....* the best mood is one of tranquil waiting...refraining from any conscious, controllable use of the brain. Letting its lower and more ancient centers take over and handle the job. Only in the absence of intellect in positive action shall we achieve painless childbirth[79].

Marilyn Moran agrees it doesn't take obstetrical skill to give birth:

> Childbirth is a normal, womanly, physiological function. What's more, it is a genital expression, and if a man and wife approach birth as a love encounter, in the same manner as they approached that other genital expression nine months earlier, then their baby will be born quite effectively.
>
> Does the nursing mother worry about the color of her milk, its composition, or the number of ounces a baby gets at a feeding? No. She just relaxes, tucks her infant close to her with her nipple in his mouth and he gets his belly filled and thrives beautifully. The foregoing are some of the details the formula manufacturers must be concerned with, however, in order to produce an acceptable substitute which can nourish a baby satisfactorily.
>
> Does the loving couple give any thought to the texture or color of the woman's cervix, or to the pH of her vaginal mucus, in order to make a baby? No. They just snuggle close and "do what comes naturally" and the next thing they know — Momma's pregnant! These are details that an obstetrician must give attention to however, in order to artificially inseminate a woman.
>
> Similarly, the birthing couple need not give a thought to the length of the contractions nor to the length of the interval between them. Neither is it necessary for a man and wife to know how many centimeters the cervix has dilated.

> As the moment of birth approaches, one's husband should not try to be a pseudo-obstetrician. He is a loving spouse and it is in this role that he has his expertise (or should!)

The Pre-and Perinatal Psychology Journal published an article written by Moran in the Spring 1993 edition entitled "Attachment or loss within marriage: The effect of the medical model of birthing on the marital bond of love."[80] The article reveals a secret many couples birthing at home in privacy have discovered: loving couples have their own personal custom-designed stress-relieving, labour-easing childbirth assistance. The things loving couples do best can help the progress of labour as well as — or better than — traditional medical intervention can. Here's how:

- Kissing can help speed and ease labour (First Base):
  > "Childbirth educators have long known that if the facial muscles of the birthing women are tense and tight the muscles in her birth canal will be too. Therefore a mother is taught to concentrate on keeping her face relaxed during labor. There is no easier way for a woman to relax her face than to get warm kisses from her husband..."
- More kissing: In addition, saliva contains androstenol, a pheromonally active substance. Pheromones are chemical messengers. Between members of a species the pheromones have a specific effect upon a target organ resulting in an alteration in sensual behavior.
- Nipple stimulation (Second Base): When you nurse a baby the nipple stimulation causes you to release oxytocin into the bloodstream. Nipple stimulation can speed up or even induce labour. This has recently been recognized and used by more progressive doctors as a safer method of induction than synthetic hormones.
- Clitoral stimulation decreases pain sensation. (Third Base)
- Sexual intercourse can help stimulate contractions, particularly if the woman has an orgasm. (Home)
- More Sex: Relaxin, a hormone which helps loosen the pubic bones for birth and soften the cervix, is present in semen. Doctors induce labour by using an extract of pig semen in gel form applied to the cervix.

Your Own Space – The Final Frontier

In a conversation with several women - each of whom had had at least one home birth - every one of us agreed we could never go back to the hospital after having the baby at home. One woman said it would be like having to go live at your parent's house again, living by their rules after having your own home.

We noticed home-birthing couples talk about "we" more: "We went upstairs; we tried some massage; we kept the baby in our bed." Hospital birth stories are more often peppered with permission than decision: "*They* let me walk around, *they* told me I could use the Jacuzzi, *they* said it was time to push, *they* let me have the baby right away."

We all agreed it was very empowering to have the baby at home. And yet, as we talked about the highlights of our births, we noticed one disturbing factor: even though we had all had lovely home births, each and every one of us had experienced something annoying, or something which ruined an otherwise perfect birth! For some, an insensitive remark by the doctor or midwife made a negative impression on the couple at a vulnerable time. Perhaps a relative or neighbour or some other attendant stayed beyond their welcome. One woman had an argument with the doctor about when and how to push. Another was rushed to deliver the placenta. Another woman was embarrassed because the midwife took pictures of her naked with baby in the tub.

The conversation made me think a lot about Marilyn Moran's idea about birth being a private affair. I remembered my son's question about being embarrassed. I tried to imagine what it would be like to give birth without any qualified attendant around. It was frightening! But deep down I had to admit to myself I always secretly hoped I would be one of those people you hear about who delivers the baby before the doctor gets there. I just knew it would never happen to me, because I have fairly long labours, with plenty of warning pain.

I closed my eyes and remembered what giving birth felt like. I vividly recalled the doctor stationed between my legs, and felt my body tense up at the memory, as I do in the dreaded Pap test. Whether in a gynecological exam, a delivery room or in my own bed, whether an obstetrician or a midwife, there was an unmistakable tension there, a self-conscious uneasiness of having anyone other than my husband in my private place, "seeing my bare bum."

Anyone other than my husband...

Then, in my mind's eye, I envisioned my husband, instead of the doctor, catching my baby. My husband — my life's partner, my bed-mate and soul mate and my partner in child-rearing — my beloved in the private place I share with him alone, receiving our child into his hands as I gave birth. Instantly my body responded to the vision as it melted into relaxation! I went from tension to tranquility: calm, composed, like coming home from a hard day at work to those welcoming arms, as I opened up and said, "aahhh..."

Why didn't I see this before? Why *wouldn't* I be more relaxed with my husband? He is the only one with whom I willingly and happily share my most private parts. Physically and emotionally, it's private territory, *our* private territory. And it's our baby, mine and his, not mine and the doctor's!

It makes sense: I know I give birth easier when I am relaxed and comfortably at ease. I am relaxed and comfortably at ease with my husband, and tense and uneasy with a doctor. Therefore, my husband is the one who should be catching the baby! The man who shares my supper table and my bathtub and my children, should share the birth — not as a bystander. Besides, he lives every day with those partly-shaven corn-rows on the backs of my legs, and has seen my bare bum.

When we discovered we were expecting #5 I was excited at the prospect of having my husband catch the baby. I asked the doctor if we could do this, and he said it would be fine with him as long as everything was going well. I was looking forward to this new dimension of childbirth.

I spent my pregnancy praying for health and strength and endurance — and patience, like any mother with toddlers. I also prayed I could have the baby a little early. "Be careful what you pray for," someone once said, "God has a sense of humour." I even prayed for a smaller baby, not because I thought it would be an easier birth, but because I wanted a baby who would look like a baby. I tend to have big, fat babies who look older than they are.[i] When you have a four-month-old wearing 18-month-size clothes, people don't think, "Wow! Look at the healthy breastfed child," they think, "That kid doesn't act like a normal one-year-old. What a moron."

So God, in His delightful sense of humour, answered my prayers in full.

One afternoon, when I was 36 weeks pregnant, I told Bert how happy and excited I was to know he was going to be catching the baby. Wouldn't it be nice if we were all alone when the baby was born, just like Marilyn Moran's book had said?

"Don't you dare!" Bert warned. "I'd be too scared."

But within 24 hours, Bert caught his own baby, all alone.

In case you think I am the most confident person in the world, let me assure you, I have the same worries and fears as everyone else. It's funny how you can forget all about the pain of childbirth after the

---

[i] I've wondered if I had gestational diabetes, which can result in larger babies, but I never had a glucose tolerance test. What I don't know hasn't hurt me.

baby is born… but next time you are pregnant, and realize you have to face birth again, it all comes back to you...

What if I can't handle the pain? What if something goes wrong? What if I really have just been "lucky" and my luck runs out and Something Terrible happens? What if my baby is ill and they rush me to the hospital and accuse me of being irresponsible for having a home birth, and take my baby away and charge me with child abuse and put me in jail and take my children away and put them in a foster home and only let me see them on court-ordered supervised visits?

Home Alone

A sharp cramp woke me out of a sound sleep. It took a minute for me to become aware enough to realize it was a contraction! A strong, powerful contraction! I got up and went to the bathroom and noticed bloody mucous. I was in labour! *How could this be happening*, I thought, *I'm not due until March 15th. It's the middle of February. And I'm usually a few days late.*

Only then did I remember my water had broken the past Sunday, five days earlier. *How could I have forgotten?* When I had felt water trickling I had been concerned, but decided the best thing to do was go to bed and just wait and see what would happen, since leaking waters can sometimes seal up on their own. But nothing happened, and I completely forgot about it. I hadn't told the doctor or even Bert about the leaking waters. *OOPS! Hadn't we had intercourse this week too? Isn't that risky?*

I thought I'd do the same this time, go to bed and forget about the mucous plug for now. But I kept getting shivers, coming in waves like contractions. Didn't I get the same shivering with some of my other labours after the water broke? I didn't want to wake Bert up so I got out of bed and went into the kitchen where I could walk around, as I usually like to do in labour. I grabbed a dust-mop and dusted the kitchen floor as I walked around and around and around the table.

And I prayed. "Lord, I know You have always taken good care of me and I know You answer prayers. This baby is too early. Should I go to the hospital this time? Should I be in the care of experts? Will my baby need intensive care?"

Now I can't say I had the experience like some have, of hearing the voice of the Lord speaking directly to them, but what I experienced was a calm contentment, an assurance, a fore-knowledge everything would be OK; serenity in a peacefulness beyond words. *It's going to be all right.*

Who was I to argue with God? I was assured it would be all right. What could I do but give thanks and praise as I walked and paced around the house, labouring in the moonlight.

I wanted it dark as I walked around and around the kitchen, dust-mop in hand, praising God. The only light was the glow from the tube light on the back of the stove. I checked the clock to see how often the contractions were coming, and counted how many long, slow breaths I took during the contraction to measure their duration.

Before I knew it, two tranquil hours had passed, the floor was cleaner than it had been in weeks, and the contractions were lasting about 15 long, slow, relaxing breaths, which I guessed must have been about two minutes. It started to really hurt, and again I spoke to the Lord.

"*Lord, this hurts! Jesus, You came to earth as a man. You never had a baby. You don't know what it is to suffer like this*!" (I get a little cranky in labour, even at God!)

And again, in a wordless answer to my prayer, I saw in my mind a vision of Jesus. I saw His feet nailed to a wooden beam, spikes piercing through the sensitive nerves of His hands, the flesh on His back ripped open and bleeding from being flogged, gasping for breath as he hung, bleeding to death. *You think I don't know what it is to suffer?*

My throat felt tight and tears burned my eyes. *Forgive me Lord!*

Compared to crucifixion a few little ol' labour pains didn't seem to amount to much any more. I made a pot of coffee for Bert and woke him at 4:00 am with the words, "You better start thinking of a name for this baby. It's going to be born today!"

Incredibly, I had just collected some of the things we needed for the birth the day before: just a few old towels and a new shoelace we would use to tie the cord. I sent Bert down to the basement to get a box of baby clothes. They were musty, so we sorted out some of the things we might need first, like receiving blankets, undershirts, and little nightgowns, and started a load of laundry. It was almost 5:00 in the morning when we called the doctor to let him know we were in labour.

We put a new vinyl tablecloth on the kitchen table (the cheap Wal-Mart kind) so we could use the old one on the floor next to the bed to protect the carpet, and then we were done. Nothing else needed for the birth but the doctor.

I let out a sigh of satisfaction. Our little 'nest' was ready, the laundry was started, and the doctor was on his way. Physically, mentally, spiritually, I was ready. I set out to do a few more laps around the kitchen table, but instead of walking, I leaned across the table, put my head down on the stiff, strong-smelling new vinyl tablecloth, and to my surprise, moaned like a moose.

Bert recognized the familiar sound meant. I was in transition. He glanced anxiously toward the window, hoping to see the lights of the doctor's car approaching. I was at a dreadful point where I wasn't sure I could handle the pain, and didn't think I could take it any longer. I tried to sit, stood up, squatted down, and stood again. *Ten contractions*, I told myself, *ten contractions like this, and the transition phase should be over. I can handle ten. I can do this.*

Ungh! Another contraction brought another loud grunting moan. I leaned on the table and Bert rubbed my lower back, pushing hard, counter-pressure against the pressure from the baby on the inside. The grunting turned to gasping as hard labour left me breathing like I was making the final few steps of a steep mountain climb. *Nine! Nine more to go. I can do this.*

Josh, age 11, woke when he heard my moose call. It was just after five o'clock in the morning, so we told him everything was OK, I was just in labour, and to go back to bed. Bert went to the window again, hoping to see the doctor's car approaching, but there was nothing but darkness and a cold wind blowing snow around the streetlights. He followed me to the bedroom where everything was ready for the birth.

UNGH! Another powerful contraction and my hips felt as if there were some giant internal vice pushing them apart. I wrapped my arms around Bert's neck and this time, held my breath. It seemed less painful. *Eight!*

Standing beside the bed, in the light of the lamp, I held on to Bert's neck, panting lightly as I recovered from the strength and awesome power of the contraction. Suddenly an idea hit me, remembering something I read in Marilyn Moran's book. "Kiss me!" I gasped.

"Huh?"

"I want you to *kiss* me." Bert gave me a polite peck on the lips.

"No! KISS ME!" I demanded, grabbing him by the face. One big slurpy delicious kiss and I felt something incredible happening deep inside.

"You're pushing!" he said accusingly, "Aren't you!"

"No-o-o" I grunted." I - don't - think - so!"

"Stop pushing!!" Bert pleaded frantically, "Wait till the doctor gets here!" I ignored him, basking in the incredible sensation of the baby sliding down into the birth canal, with no straining on my part.

"Don't push! Don't do this!" he pleaded.

"Will you just shut up? It's all right!" *What's he so upset about,* I wondered. *I've been talking to God all night and it's going to be all right. What's his problem?*

I glanced at the waterbed, decided it was too soft for giving birth, and slid down from Bert's arms to sit on the floor where the tablecloth was protecting the carpet, and leaned back against the side of the bed.

"Oh God!" cried Bert, lifting my nightgown, "There's the head!"

And here comes the rest of it, I thought, as my body opened up and released — a wonderful, earthy sensation — and the baby slid into Bert's hands.

"What do I do? What do I do?" Bert said nervously, as he caught the slippery little baby. "What do I do? What do I do?" he fretted as he placed the baby in my arms, just as the baby peed, squirting my leg. "What do I do?" Bert asked the air as he grabbed a towel from the pile I had placed by the bed and put it over the baby to keep him warm. "What do I do? What do I do?" he chanted fretfully, as he was *doing* exactly what needed to be done.

The baby was already crying, and so was I – crying tears of joy and squealing with delight in the high-pitched helium voice newly-delivered women use, and laughing out loud. One of the children woke up to the excited squeals and laughter, and thinking there was a tickling contest going on in the bedroom, came in to join the fun. Suddenly the atmosphere was like Christmas morning, as they ran excitedly room to room, waking everyone up to see the wonderful surprise!

Bert was on the phone frantically trying to get hold of the doctor, who, assuming there was plenty of time, had gone to his office in town for supplies. I told Bert to calm down, for crying out loud! After all, the baby was OK, I was OK, *everything was OK!* What was the worry? I'd *told* him it was going to be all right, after all!

When the cord turned white and lifeless, I tied it with the shoelace and cut it with my good hairdressing scissors, so I could get up off the floor. I was tidying up some wet towels off the floor with the baby in one arm and my end of the cord still dangling between my legs when the doctor appeared in the doorway. He put his hands on his hips, observed the scene, and shook his head. "Don't they ever let you rest?" he laughed.

The doctor said the baby was perfectly healthy, at about five and a half pounds. He reprimanded us for tying off the cord a little too long. (Big deal, the cord fell off in three days, all six inches of it.) The main concern, he said, would be if the baby experienced any breathing difficulty. Like a mother kangaroo, I kept my little joey in a pouch: I wore him in a cloth sling all day, and at night he slept on my chest. My body became — or rather continued to be — his incubator, regulating his temperature and his breathing by the warmth and movement of his mother's body.

There are other subtle factors coming into play when we give birth in the presence of others, which we fail to realize have an effect on the marriage relationship I noticed a strong fatherly protectiveness Bert had for the baby, much more so than he had with the others. I also saw him many times holding the baby, speaking softly, proudly saying, "I was the first one to ever touch you!"

I felt great. I was on an emotional high which lasted for months. Even the afterpains were mild. On the second day after birth we entertained friends for the evening. Surprisingly I was not the least tired and there was no soreness at all. On the third day we showed up for church as usual to everyone's surprise. By the sixth day the lochial flow had even stopped!

And on the seventh day we rested... or at least that's what we told the kids we were doing in the bedroom.

And it was very good.

CHAPTER 12

The "X"-(Rated) Files

"I present unassisted childbirth not as a way childbirth *should* be done, but rather as a way it *can* be done."

Laura Kaplan Shanley
Unassisted Childbirth

You might need a cold shower after reading this chapter. Pretend you have a headache and go into your room to read. Hide the book inside a copy of *Good Housekeeping* Magazine.

Skinny Dipping in the Moonlight

Some people will only swim in nice clean pools. They would never take the risk of swimming anywhere except where they know the water has been chlorinated, the lifeguard is watching, and they can touch bottom.

If a typical hospital birth is like swimming laps in an indoor heated, chlorinated pool, home birth is like skinny-dipping in the moonlight. They each have their benefits, but pools-only people don't know what they're missing.

Have you ever gone skinny-dipping on a dark night with the one you love? In the darkness, you hurry down to the water's edge, slip off your clothes, and toss them to the shore. Shivering with the initial chill in the water, you cling to each other's naked skin, the goosebumps rough under your hands. Before too long, you get used to the water, and you start across the river.

How wonderful the water feels against your naked skin, flowing through your hair, around your breasts. Naked and uninhibited in the dark you open your legs wide and enjoy the coolness of refreshing water between your legs.

The deep water lifts you and you feel the power of the current pulling you from the shore. Stronger and stronger flows the current, and you find it hard to catch your breath. But unhindered by the restrictive swimsuits, and free from the watchful eyes of others, you make this journey together, treading water while you embrace, happily anticipating the opposite shore. You are oblivious to the passing time as the cold water, the strength of the current, and the excitement of the journey fills your consciousness.

You begin to tire, and the work of swimming in the current takes all your concentration. You feel so alive, so aware in all your senses: the smell of the damp air, the sound of the gentle splash of your arms pushing through the water, bubbles rippling along your naked belly. You notice the strength of your own arms and legs as they propel you forward through the current, each stroke bringing you closer, closer to the opposite shore. You can see the dark outline of the trees as you draw nearer. Suddenly, to your surprise, you feel gritty sand at your feet. A few more strokes and you touch the bottom! You have made it! You feel wonderful! Exhilarated! Triumphant!

The lap swimmers meet you later on the shore. "What did you do that for?" they ask, "That was dangerous. You could have got just as good a workout in our nice pool with the lifeguards on duty."

Cultural Expectations

Our culture influences our belief system, and so our ideas about birth, babies, and breastfeeding are dictated by our civilization. Culture also dictates what is considered "normal." For example, in our culture it is "normal" for women to wean from the breast after a 3-6 months, but among the "!Kung" tribe in Africa, it is quite normal for children to nurse for six or eight years![81] In a Brazilian tribe, a researcher[82] noticed it was simply a matter of course for children to witness their parents making love since families sleep together — a practice our culture believes is not good for children. In our culture sex is private. Childbirth is not.

While the same organs of procreation are used both to conceive and give birth to a baby, one is a private, loving encounter between two people; the other is attended by strangers. One event demands privacy; the other demands observation. We fail to see any connection between the two events, guarding the privacy of one event, while insisting on attendance at the other. Look at the contrast: The first procreative event happens best when couples are undistracted and free from interruption, where they enjoy the sensations freely and uninhibited usually in a dark, private place. The second event occurs in a brightly lit room, surrounded by strangers, where sensations are chemically dulled or otherwise avoided as much as possible and everyone is completely covered — with the exception of the woman's private parts.

Imagine for a moment you live in an alternate universe where these two aspects of procreation are switched. Imagine on your wedding night culture dictated that your friends, parents, and in-laws had to monitor your progress. Or that a doctor was required to supervise the actual consummation of marriage for legal documentation. Either way, someone will be present throughout the consummation. There will be bright lights and people are entitled to barge in unannounced at any time. They might wish to inspect your bodies to make sure things are happening as they are supposed to. They will give you encouragement. Absurd, isn't it! You'd be so inhibited! Could you and your spouse manage under those conditions? Or would you need some pharmaceutical assistance to complete the task?

Yet when the same sexual organs that received the seed of conception are now releasing the finished product in childbirth, how can we think we aren't equally inhibited by the presence of outsiders at this event?

This brings to mind another medical procedure involving something being extracted from the organs of reproduction: sperm donation. In a scene from the movie *Forget Paris*, Billy Crystal's character has to give his sperm for artificial insemination. He is shown to a private room with a television and a stack of adult magazines and videos, to help him, well... finish the job. If sperm donation is a medical procedure (like childbirth) why don't they spray him with antiseptic and make him lie on a table under a bright light draped in sterile sheets, whereupon the gloved, gowned, and masked staff can collect his donation in a sterile container?

We accept it as a matter of course that several strangers will be present to witness what is ultimately the culmination of the sex act. To imagine childbirth now in the same sense as lovemaking stretches the limits of our cultural taboos. To compare the two is unthinkable! It crosses the boundaries of our society's moral thinking.

Laura Kaplan Shanley, author of *Unassisted Childbirth* writes:

> Most women in this culture have been led to believe they are incapable of delivering their own babies. Even most feminists, who look back in horror to the days when women were told they must rely on others (generally men) for their emotional and financial support, still do not hesitate in labor to turn themselves over to a person of "authority." The notion that women are self-reliant, independent, competent human beings has not, at this point in time, been fully applied to the act of giving birth. Childbirth—an event that should ideally reinforce a woman's sense of power and

> autonomy—has now become a painful, dangerous ordeal that often ends up reinforcing the belief she is indeed a helpless, dependent child herself.[83]

One wonders what effect there might be upon mankind if men felt frightened, powerless, and in need of assistance for their most basic procreative attempts.

The Sexuality of Childbirth

The first time I got a hint of the sexuality of birth was the moment my second son was born. My first baby had been removed from my body during a cesarean section while I was asleep; it was a surgical event. The second baby was born vaginally with no medication. I noticed something surprisingly sexual happened, but I couldn't find the words to describe it. It was a thrilling moment of familiarity and connection — a sense of completion and yet beginning.

After this exhilarating experience I often asked women excitedly, "Did you get to touch the baby as soon as it was born?" Many of them would say, yes, they did—just as soon as they cleaned the baby off. Then I knew they had missed the most incredible part.

Under the bright lights, covered by sterile sheets, amidst the stranger's eyes peering over their masks, I experienced something profoundly sexual that gloved hands would not notice. When the baby was laid on my belly and I reached out and touched him, there was immediately a déjà vu moment of recognition… a feeling of something familiar. Giving birth was new to me, but this sensation was not! It's very difficult to describe without sounding vulgar… the hot, sticky-wet, throbbing, pulsating flesh had just come out of me, covered in a creamy white stuff... just like… well... *just like when the baby was started nine months earlier!*

Do the gloved hands recognize this? Do they hide it from us on purpose to separate women from a full understanding of their sexuality? Or do they just cover it up in distaste?

If something sexual truly *is* happening and the medical people meddle or stand around and watch, it's embarrassing for us and downright vulgar for them. There can only be two ways of dealing with the problem. First, they could allow parents their privacy. Staff members would be there in case of emergency. It sounds like an ideal solution. But then there would be a shift in power. Parents would be in control, staff would be there to serve.

The second option keeps the medical people in control. This is accomplished by trying to mask, hide or remove the sexuality of birth.

Robbie Davis-Floyd comments:

> So effective are hospital routines at masking the intense sexuality of birth that most women today are not even aware of birth's sexual nature. For example, stimulation of the laboring woman's breasts and clitoris has been proven to be extremely effective in strengthening labor, yet is utterly taboo in most hospitals, where the synthetic hormone Pitocin is administered intravenously instead. The routine performance of episiotomy is another excellent example of the desexualization of birth in the hospital: an effective alternative recommended by many midwives is perineal massage with warm olive oil, far too overtly sexual a procedure for most obstetricians. Through Pitocin and episiotomies, sterile gowns and sheets, enemas and pubic shaves, anesthesia and orange antiseptic, the intense and potentially ecstatic sexuality of birth is consistently and effectively masked.[84]

Fear of Womanhood

In the early 1900's it was understood that men needed sex and women were to submit to it to fulfill their marital duty. A woman's ability to achieve orgasm wasn't understood, partly because it was not expected and partly because it was subjective. The shuddering, ecstatic sensation women occasionally experienced during intercourse was thought to be conception occurring.[85] Women didn't mind submitting to intercourse, but only a tramp (or weirdo) would admit to ever *liking* it. It was expected to hurt a lot the first time. Brides were terrified of the wedding night because of the pain and the blood they anticipated.

The result of the sexual union of course leads to an even greater fear: childbirth. We are terrified of the pain and the blood, especially the first time. We recognize it is not as bad the second time and those brave enough to have more than two are sometimes even looking forward to the big event. But only a weirdo (tramp?) would admit she *liked* giving birth!

Similarly, most women begin breastfeeding to fulfill their motherly duty to the child. But occasionally, the tender skin of the nipples, not accustomed to the stimulation, can become cracked and bleed. Upon hearing this, many women are terrified of breastfeeding because of the pain and the blood.[i]

Some of us weirdos actually admit to liking breastfeeding, tramps that we are. Not only does it feel good physically, with the little mouth rhythmically milking the nipple; many women also enjoy a deeper understanding of their femininity, experience a profound expression of their womanliness, and luxuriate in a warm, intimate

---

[i] Many pre-pubescent girls are also afraid of menstruation because of the anticipated pain and blood.

relationship with their babies. Breastfeeding should be enjoyable. If it's not, there's a problem.

A woman who enjoys sex is not considered a weirdo or a slut any more. We have a positive attitude and expect sex to be enjoyable. If it's not, there's a problem.

We have to identify what's causing the fear of childbirth, because like frightened virgin brides, some of us are so are so afraid of experiencing pain, we choose to not feel anything at all.

Going All the Way

Marilyn Moran's *Birth and the Dialogue of Lov*e "goes all the way" claiming if birth is indeed a sexual experience, it ought to be accomplished in the privacy of a couple's bedroom. Marilyn felt that if birth is sexual, then having a doctor deliver your baby is adultery, and a midwife-attended delivery likened to a lesbian affair. I wonder what Moran would say about Patricia Carter and Laura Shanley who chose to do it alone!

Laura Kaplan Shanley writes:

> My husband was present when I gave birth to my first and second babies, and I thoroughly enjoyed his company. However, on subsequent births, I chose to be alone because I viewed it as my personal challenge. It gave me the opportunity to depend completely on myself, and I found that indeed I could.[86]

The daughter of a medical doctor, Shanley chose to give birth at home unassisted because her research and understanding led her to conclude intervention made birth more difficult. Like Carter, Shanley believed she would be better off getting in touch with her more primitive self than seeking professional assistance.

> [T]he majority of people in intellectually developed societies are both psychologically and physically unhealthy. Because they are unaware of the existence of the inner self, they are unable to utilize the constant help and guidance that is available to them. Animals, on the other hand, have little sense of themselves as individuals, but they intuitively avail themselves of this guidance.
>
> The tribal woman, in a sense, has a consciousness that lies between that of the animal and that of the modern Western woman. Her births are successful for several reasons. She has not yet developed beliefs in fear, shame, and guilt, and therefore is free from their devastating consequences. In addition to this, like the cat in the closet, she is generally left alone. This privacy not only allows her body to perform its task easily because it is unhampered by outside intervention, it also allows her to psychologically reconnect with her inner self. The inner self speaks to her—just as it does to the Western woman—through her dreams, impulses, and intuition. The difference is, she listens.[87]

Moran, however, believes a woman actually has a real physical need for her husband's presence during childbirth, as pheromones pass from the man to the woman to aid her labour.

> When I gave birth at home, I was sitting on the floor on sterilized padding with my knees drawn up, as my husband knelt at my side with his arms around me. At the very end of labor, I came out of a dozing state and found he had lowered his head and the side of his face was just an inch in front of mine. Staring momentarily into the pores at the side of his nose and mouth, the thought flashed through my mind, "My, what big pores you have!" With that I was aware of a great pressure at my perineum. Then the pressure was gone. I asked, "What's that?" My husband replied, "The head."
>
> Thereupon, I threw my head back and ecstatically cried out, "And there's the body!" as I felt a swirling sensation from my groin. Looking down I saw the baby between my legs squirming and moving his arms about.
>
> I did not smell anything. But I strongly suspect that my husband, my partner in the nine month conjugal love dialogue, emitted a specific pheromone through the pores of his face which had a beneficial effect on me in accomplishing the task at hand in a way that no obstetrician nor anyone else could have done. Men's pores around the nose and mouth are larger than women's. There is a good reason for this. Nothing happens by chance in nature.[88]

Similarly, Ina May Gaskin's book *Spiritual Midwifery* shows many photos of smiling couples kissing during labour and birth, and in some pictures the husband is seen fondling his wife's breasts. Gaskin encourages "smooching" to help the labour progress.[89]

> "When someone says, "I love you" and means it, it opens up his throat—it literally does it. And when the throat opens up so does the cervix. I've been checking a lady's dilation at the same time she'd say that, and I could feel a distinct difference in her tissue, in how stretchy she was, that was exactly synchronous with her saying, "I love you." It made me really understand that words are vibrations and that some combinations of words have greater power than others. "I love you" is very strong.[90]

Territorial Rights

There are numerous assaults to the marriage relationship when you give birth in the presence of others, subtle factors we don't generally consider but factors which may cause unrest in some couples. For example: How does a husband really feel when another man stands between his wife's legs, touching her in places she should reserve for him and him alone? How does it affect him, if only on a subconscious level, when he stands at his wife's head in the delivery room while the medical staff stand between her legs? What does his deepest gut instinct tell him about the situation? What does it say about his manhood, allowing this to happen to his woman? How does he feel about his wife, exposing herself to others?

Picture yourself in labour, nine months pregnant and huge. Your ankles are swollen, you're wearing a Hospital Patient Uniform (which doesn't quite cover the new dimension of your rear) and your mucous plug is sliding down your leg. Oh, look! A couple of slim, pretty, young nurses enter the room and hover near you in their crisp clean uniforms, their hair pinned neatly in place, with a scent of light perfume and a fresh coat of lipstick applied. In contrast, you have been in labour for 17 hours, are sweaty, hungry, tired and miserable. You have stretch marks, and your belly button is sticking out so far you found lint in it that's been buried for four years.

Next the handsome young intern comes in. It's his turn to check your dilation. Your husband watches as you spread your legs for the handsome dude. He notices you haven't been up to spreading your legs much for *him*, lately.

You have blood on your thighs, and as he examines you, you accidentally pass wind, in the presence of both men.

Why can't hospitals grant you privacy behind a locked door? With the assurance of privacy, the security of available medicine if it becomes necessary, and the safety of available technology, couples should be allowed to labour in respected privacy, knowing help is just a call-bell away. Perhaps this option isn't allowed because undoubtedly some couples would realize they could just as easily have stayed home.

Ultimately, this would eliminate the problem of women arriving at hospitals and being turned away due to a lack of beds. The low-risk women would be birthing at home, leaving beds available to the high-risk women who truly need them.

Birth as a Climax

Patricia Carter believed painless birth enhances the parents love for each other, even if the woman gives birth without her husband presence.

> "... down thru the centuries, Man has subconsciously thought sex ought by rights to be a pleasant thing. Subconsciously he has felt frustrated because he has the human wish to bring naught but joy in love to his mate. Not willingly would he be a party to her pain. The shadow of her martyrdom beats like distant drumbeats and melancholy rain to mar the blissful sweets of Love. Man wants to love her freely, and for her freely to return his love. Freely, without that painful shadow hovering. And when he hears her screams in childbirth, he vows that never again will he put her thru such suffering. And when again the inevitable enchantment has worked its magic and she has again conceived, he feels like a puppet driven

> by a power greater than himself, and he is hurt because in spite of himself he has hurt her again. And sometimes, way down deep, there is a smoldering anger that despite all he can do in laying at her feet the fruits of his daily toil and the sweat of his brow, there is still this haunting sense of guilt for pain which he cannot prevent. The unconscious struggle within the depths of his being is bodied forth, alas, in irritation, or he takes refuge in inhibiting his desires in disinterestedness, in order to protect himself from the silent reproaches.
>
> "They are barred from true Friendship which is the grace of love. Alas, in too many cases the Beauty, the exquisiteness of the Love they knew in their youth when the Price of pain was distant, and not a keen and known reality, has vanished. The Oneness is gone. She stands alone in her needless pain, he in his needless guilt. For pain is loneliness. Guilt is loneliness. Only gladness can be truly shared.
>
> "This truth was brought home to me in the letters I received. The curious difference in the use of the personal pronoun was significant. Those letters from women who had known only pain in childbirth are filled with the singular form. "I had my child" "I suffered" "The doctor told me" "My baby." Always, always singular. For pain is singular. The letters from women who had had relatively painless births in naturalness wrote, "We had our baby." "We had no trouble." "The doctor told us." Not "My baby," but "Our baby". A sharing. One seldom hears a man or woman say "My honeymoon." It is generally "our honeymoon" when they reminisced. Gladness is plural.
>
> Pain is a wedge between Man and Woman. Guilt is a wedge between them. Gladness is a bridge uniting them.[91]

Lynn Griesemer, author of *Unassisted Childbirth - An Act of Love* comments on privacy:

> "A couple who births a child in the same privacy in which they conceived the child strengthens their union and is more likely to achieve sexual fulfillment. Making love should be a private, personal affair and the ultimate result of that joining together, birthing a baby, should be done in a modest setting. It is the most healthy scenario in achieving femininity and masculinity. The presence of a midwife inhibits this achievement and detracts from the true experience of childbirth at its core element. Childbirth is and should be approached as a sexual experience. Since I would not want a midwife present while making love with my husband, I do not want a midwife present while having a baby with my husband."[92]

Griesemer, like many others, believes there is more to home birth than just being in your own bed:

> There have been many accounts of pleasurable birth, more often by women who give birth privately. That means outside the hospital, with only her spouse present, or in some cases, alone.

> Birth at home in the presence of midwives or other support people has also enabled women to give birth pleasurably. The reason for this is that birth is sexual and sensual and that a certain level of modesty is crucial for a pleasurable birth. Hospital births are more often described as tolerable rather than pleasurable.[93]

Catherine Young, Editor of *The Compleat Mother* Magazine published a collection of joyful, uplifting birth stories from the magazine in a booklet called *Birth Joy*. For the pregnant woman who is nervous about her upcoming delivery—and who isn't?!—it is very reassuring to fill your thoughts with delightfully different birth stories in contrast to the usual doctor-managed deliveries.

> He was born at home, without midwives, because they are institutionalized, and don't like such ideas. There was my husband, myself, and God. It was wonderful, magical, and sensual. When I pushed my baby out it was a generous orgasm.
>
> *-Gabriela A., Argentina*
>
> I went into labour in the night. I only wanted to be alone, so I got up and did a little dance-walk all over our house. The night was quiet and I felt like a giant goddess woman rolling my pelvis with each wonderful contraction...
>
> I suddenly had an overwhelming urge to get on the toilet. I felt better as soon as I was there. James came in and asked if he should call the midwife...
>
> James was running past as my baby's head was gently born into my waiting hand. I never pushed and there was no pain... I asked [James] if he wanted to see his baby's head. He chuckled and said, "Yeah, right." I stood up and lifted up my shirt. My husband's eyes got enormous! The next contraction came and out gushed my beautiful baby boy...
>
> My son weighed 10 lbs., 4 ounces. He was 23 inches long. I did not tear or even feel pain with his birth. I made love with God's help, deep in the night and am blessed by my experience.
>
> *-Natalie B., Texas*
>
> The lights were out. I bathed in water and darkness. I felt frightened, a little, but I also trusted my body to do the work it had to do. An hour passed. It wasn't pain, exactly. More of a passion that swept over me, over and over and over. My mouth opened and shut in unison with the rhythmic stretching, stretching of my cervix.
>
> Open, open, my mouth stretched in wordless song. I needed nothing; I was in awe of my body.
>
> Open, open, and suddenly, aaaaaaah. My baby slid down, through, and there, ready to pass into the world. My husband came, fetching a receiving blanket. I left the bath then, and entered the room our son was conceived in. I stood by our bed, ready.
>
> Another push, then a dark, damp lock of hair came. The head, oh, beautiful red, and shortly, his whole body passed into my husband's hands.

> Smiling, laughing, tears, and whoops of joy. The man who shares my bed and table and life passed me our child. I raised my infant to my breast, and kissed his blessed head a hundred times. I licked him and marveled at his darling fat. We laughed at his large, red balls. We celebrated his first pee. The earth moved.
>
> *-Kelly Williams, Orangeville, Ontario*

In Childbirth Alternatives Quarterly, Davis-Floyd described her sexual birth experience:

> "I really think the issue of clitoral stimulation in labor needs to be openly discussed. I can't believe that I had to try to hide from the midwives and everyone else present what I was asking Robert to do - I mean, there I was totally naked, legs wide open, getting ready to push a baby out - but somehow for Robert to rub my clitoris was shameful. He was very embarrassed, but I loved it - it felt wonderful to have a little bit of pleasure right smack in the middle of all that pain. Maybe it's not that it's so shameful, but it's simply a very intensely private thing. And maybe the solution is not to have so many people around, or to have the strength to ask them to leave for private times."

Jeanine Parvati-Baker gives another description of the intense sexual nature of birth as she experienced it:

> I feel the baby come down. The sensation is ecstatic. I had prepared somewhat for this being as painful as my last delivery had been. Yet this time the pulse of birth feels wonderful! I am building up to the birth climax after nine months of pleasurable foreplay. With one push the babe is in the canal. The next push brings him down, down, into that space just before orgasm when we women know how God must have felt creating this planet.
>
> The water supports my birth outlet. I feel connected to the mainland, to my source. These midwife hands know just what to do to support the now crowning head, coming so fast. How glad I am for all those years of orgasms! Slow orgasms, fast ones, those which build and subside and peak again and again. That practice aids my baby's gentle emergence so that he doesn't spurt out too quickly. He comes, as do I.

Lester D. Hazell, in *Commonsense Childbirth*:

> "It should be noted here that a few women experience labor and delivery as an intensely sexual happening. In a socially permissive atmosphere, some will want to masturbate or be masturbated repeatedly to orgasm during first stage and may experience second stage as a series of orgasms with each contraction. Birth comes as one big orgasm. Not all women find birth directly sexual, though for most it has some sexual overtones. It is probably these sexual overtones, unrecognized, that cause some women to fall in love with their obstetricians when the husband has not been an active participant in the birth.
>
> "... life produces changes in our sexuality. The pregnancy cycle produces particularly massive ones. Failure to be in touch with

> these changes, to accept them, and to find new, better ways of expressing our sexuality can lead to a terrible sense of worsening. We are sexual beings from birth to death, at whatever age the latter occurs. Women are different from men and express their sexuality through the menstrual cycles, through intercourse, through masturbation, through pregnancy, labor, delivery, and breastfeeding... Both sexes are capable of experiencing a far wider ability to be sexual, and pregnancy offers the chance to grow, to dissolve old barriers, and to become more authentic people."[94]

Indeed, the very idea of childbirth being pleasurable stretches our thinking and beliefs. One woman said comparing the horrendous pain of childbirth with sexual pleasure suggests masochism. Others find it merely distasteful.

Laura O'Banion boldly reveals the true source of our aversion:

> "since it was supposed that only the penis (or an analogue thereof) was capable of providing sexual satisfaction, the penis-analogue in childbirth must be — the child itself!"[95]

It seems the Ultimate Orgasm occurs when the man's seed, having been planted in the woman, tended, and fully ripened, is ejaculated back to him in a joyful harvest of new life. Just as you can have great sex away from your own familiar bed, like at a hotel, I believe you could have a great birth in the hospital, if you were granted the same privacy

Thawing Out Your Frigidity

For the prudish types who are so afraid of naughty sex they act as if all sexuality is dirty, I have some comments.

According to the bible, wives are to submit themselves to their husbands. And oh, how we can struggle with that! But we learn — often the hard way — that it is in submission our joy is released. Submission means to yield to another. Submitting yourself to the needs of the newborn baby, instead of trying to control his feeding pattern, frees you to fully enjoy the baby. When lovemaking, it is only when a woman submits to the sensations she discovers ecstasy. Also in childbirth, submit yourself to the sensations, and enjoy the ride. Easy childbirth is not about taking total control; it's about total surrender.

In a seminar given at a La Leche League Conference, Dr. Carolyn Rawlings said that when God plugged the cervix during pregnancy to protect the baby from germs, He could have just as easily plugged the vagina and made intercourse impossible. But He left the vagina open for a reason. God's design also put a clitoris right by the vagina. Why? It's only known purpose is for sexual pleasure. Use it! Orgasm brings strong contractions, toning the uterus. Enjoy it!

God put hormones in semen called prostaglandins, which help soften the cervix. Let it!

Lovemaking, pregnant or not, brings you closer emotionally, helps you physically communicate with each other and deepens your intimate understanding of each other's bodies. This is especially important for <u>your husband</u> at this time. Enjoy sex throughout your pregnancy, and don't be afraid of lovemaking it in your last month. Some doctors don't think it's a good idea in the last few weeks claiming a higher risk of infection, or a risk of premature labour. But I'll bet in your marriage vows, you heard, "What God hath joined together, let no man separate." Let them do without; you go ahead and enjoy the heightened sensations if God says so.

Your husband can be your love slave. The better he knows what you want now, the better he will know what you need when you are in labour. Besides, that's his job. He has to submit too. "The husband should fulfill his marital duty to his wife, and likewise the wife to her husband. The wife's body does not belong to her alone but also to her husband. In the same way, the husband's body does not belong to him alone but also to his wife. Do not deprive each other..." [i]

God said so, so do as you're told. Remember, God told Adam and Eve to be fruitful, and multiply, and *fill* the earth. That was quite an assignment. They must have been busy.

Dr. Rawlings also said there is more blood flow to the genitals during pregnancy, so the woman is in a heightened state of arousal. Many women experience orgasm for the first time during pregnancy, or become multi-orgasmic for the first time.

On the down side of this, sometimes - especially toward the end of your pregnancy - you may feel like your innards are going to fall on the floor after you make love. Restrict lovemaking to bedtime or a Sunday afternoon when you can stay in bed for a couple of hours afterwards. Or, if you have older children, I personally believe this is why cartoons are scheduled for Saturday mornings.

In the Penthouse

By Alena James

Reprinted with permission[96]

Rob had been waiting for this day for months.

Today, he and Dianne were finally going to do it! Their first time! They were both excited and a little nervous. What would people

---

[i] 1 Corinthians 7:3-5

think of them? What would their parents do, if they knew what was about to happen? They'd be furious, of course.

"I guess I'm ready," said Dianne, a little apprehensively. Rob smiled. He had been waiting a long time for this. To think, Dianne had saved this for him alone. Rob could hardly wait. His heart pounded in eager anticipation. Easy, he told himself, this might be difficult for Dianne.

It seemed like ages that he had been waiting, longing for the day Dianne would be ready to go through with it. Finally, she was ready! This was it! This would be the fulfillment of their love, the ultimate bond to cement their relationship to each other.

Dianne prepared the bed, making it with fresh clean sheets. Rob noticed she had even thought to protect the mattress with a plastic sheet. It was just like Dianne, to worry about every detail. Giggling, Dianne put a couple of towels nearby. "Just how much do you expect to bleed?" Rob teased. He put some soft music on to play.

While Dianne had been preparing the bedroom, Rob had prepared a warm, sensuous bath for her, scented with oils. Flickering candles reflected their light off the steaming water, inviting them into its soothing warmth. Slowly, Rob unbuttoned her dress and helped her into the tub, and then he undressed quickly himself and slipped in behind her. Dianne lay back against his firm, muscular chest.

Rob began to gently stroke his fingers across Dianne's forehead, then slowly down her neck, exploring her chest and lingering at her large dark nipples. He playfully pinched them and circled them with his fingers, around and around. He felt Dianne squirm, and watched with satisfaction as her nipples became erect.

"Mmmmmm," Dianne moaned softly. "Keep doing that."

Rob kept stimulating her nipples, slowly, tenderly, watching her squirm, writhing more and more. Her breathing started to come faster, and she began to rhythmically rock her pelvis, and would rub her legs together. He was enthralled, watching her, and wondered if perhaps he should ease off a bit. He didn't want to rush things.

Dianne was moaning now. She was ready! Rob stood up and dried off quickly, wrapping a towel around his waist. Holding a towel out for Dianne, he reached his strong arms around her and helped her up. She wrapped her arms around his neck, her long hair falling back as she turned her face up to meet his hungry mouth with a passionate kiss. Rob could feel her excitement, a certain tenseness in her body that excited him even more.

"Are you sure you still want to do this?" Again he teased her gently. She could only let out a low moan in answer.

Rob practically carried her to the bed, arms around each other in a flurry of kisses. Dianne lay down on her side, her arms grasping

Rob, her eyes pleading, Come to me... Rob looked with admiration at her. God, she is beautiful, he thought, his eyes drinking in the fullness of her raw beauty. She looked lovely, voluptuous, her full naked body so ripe, her lips open, panting, her arms begging for him.

Rob put his mouth on hers and kissed her deeply. His large hand gently caressed between Dianne's legs, and she spontaneously opened them, welcoming his touch. She felt slippery and swollen, her flesh pulsating with anticipation. Rob felt her trembling in his embrace. From fear or from excitement, it did not matter. They were past the point of no return, and now they would be united in a physical and emotional bond that would add a new depth and dimension to their relationship.

Aaahh, she could feel it as it entered her vagina. She gasped and held her breath. Sweat beaded on her forehead and her lip. She rolled her eyes and moaned as her most intimate part was stretched as never before. "Oh!" she cried out, "Ohhh!" Dianne took a deep breath and shuddered. She released herself, surrendering all to the overwhelming sensations in her body. Something let go deep inside of her very soul, and she lost all control, as grunts and gasps came from the depths of her very being. She clutched and grasped at Rob, pulling his hair, her toes curled and she stifled a scream. She felt as if she would split open and she cried out again.

Suddenly she felt a gush between her legs and looked down. There was Rob, on his knees between her legs, gasping with excitement, breathing hard and fast. Then she saw it: the hot naked skin was slick as it slid from the warm wetness of her body; slippery-wet from her own vagina, and coated in a creamy white substance. Her eyes bulged in surprise at the sight of this purplish mass of throbbing, pulsating flesh that had given her such amazing new sensations. It was so... big!

Rob held it in his hand, his eyes sparkling, his face beaming as never before.

"It's a BOY!" he announced, as the baby took his first breath.

CHAPTER 13

Ode to "the Toad"

The birth of my fifth baby gave me the inspiration to write this book. He was born a month premature, to an Rh-negative, previously sectioned, multiparous, overweight woman over 35 with a history of large babies, miscarriage and spotting; by an untrained, unprepared, frightened father, at home on the bedroom floor. This reads like an obstetrical nightmare, but was the best birth I had – and the most romantic thing my husband and I have ever done!

At only about five and a half pounds, the baby, who rarely opened his eyes as if he wasn't yet ready to face the world, was red, wrinkled, and ugly. We adored him. We named him Todd, but because of his strange appearance and the odd way he splayed his skinny little legs, for the first little while he carried the nickname "The Toad."

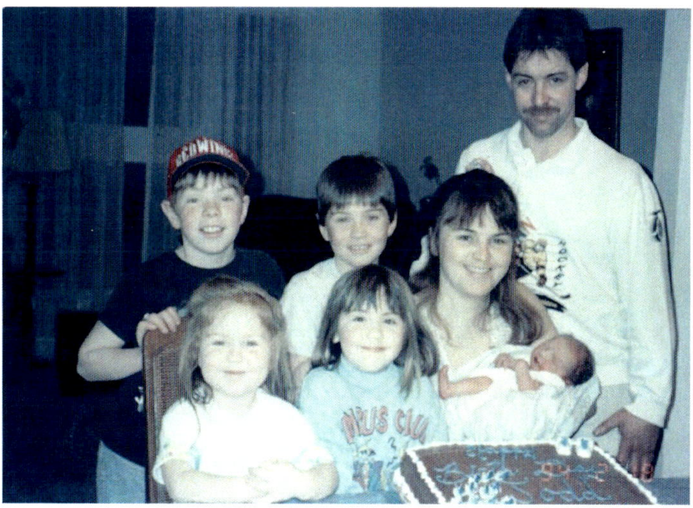

The Birth Day Party for "The Toad"

Ode to "The Toad"

Here is the story, a rhyming rendition
About our new baby, our latest addition
Who came to our household, at five in the morn
And caused quite a panic the day he was born.

He was due the next month, so I wasn't scared,
I knew there was still time for getting prepared.
Not that it takes a lot of preparing
When birthing at home (for those of us daring.)

But early one morning - the clock said two thirty -
I woke with a cramp, and Boy! Was it hurting!
That wasn't a cramp! I thought with alarm,
It's premature labour. Will it cause any harm?

Now, Bert had been out playing hockey 'til late
So reluctant to wake him, and tell him our fate,
I left him to sleep, so he hadn't a clue
That his wife was up wondering what she should do.

Should I go to the hospital? No, I think not.
They'll hook me to monitors, give me a shot,
Poke me and prod me and all of the rest.
No thanks! I'll stay home, where I feel the best.

In this situation, in such a position,
I called on the Lord, the Greatest Physician
The Author of Life, Who removed all my doubt
And I knew that in Him all things would work out.

So with God in the lead, and me praising His name
I picked up a dust-mop, and made up a game
Of timing contractions while mopping the floor.
Forget about "breathing" - I tried that before.

I paced and I mopped and talked to the Lord,
Drank raspberry tea - good for labour, I've heard,
Walked faster, breathed slower with each contraction
Enjoying the dark, and the lack of distraction.

When it got harder to deal with the pain
And I realized we still hadn't picked out a name

I woke up my husband and told him to plan
What to call our new baby, and give me a hand.

"It's four in the morning. Why are you up?"
I told him, "The coffee is made, have a cup
Then go get a box from the basement shelf
With baby clothes, diapers, and whatever else
Of the things we might need for the babe right away.
Just think! It's going to be born today!"

We started the wash, and I called the Doc
By then it was already past five o'clock.
Doctor was sleepy. He asked, "Should I hurry?"
I told him that I was OK, not to worry.

After all I had the Great Physician,
As well as Women's Intuition,
A husband who loved me, the comforts of home,
The darkness that soothed, the freedom to roam,
No bags to pack, no people to phone,
The privacy to be alone…

Much like a honeymoon, memories remain
Of those sweet moments spent before Baby came.

> Then Bert, who knows me better than anyone on earth
> Could see the subtle change in me that meant impending birth.
> I wrapped my arms around him,
> My forehead bathed in sweat,
> My breath in rasping, grunting gasps,
> The doctor not there yet!
>
> The pain seemed somehow better if I held my breath...
> "DON'T PUSH!"
> But something moved inside me...
> "Stop pushing! PLEASE!"
> "Oh SHUSH!"
> I slid down to the floor, and leaned back against the bed
> Bert knelt down right beside me. "My God! There's the head!"

Ode to the Toad

The way a flower opens and pushes forth its bloom,
A tiny little baby made his entrance in the room
His dad adeptly caught him, in spite of all his fears.
And I could hardly see him for my eyes were full of tears...

The baby was a-screaming, the second he was born.
Bert wrapped him in a towel, a soft one, frayed and worn.
I was laughing, I was crying, my heart so full of joy!
He was hot and wet and sticky, our tiny little boy.

The other children heard the fuss and entered in a horde.
Bert sterilized a shoelace and scissors for the cord.
We cuddled and we kissed and gave the babe my breast
We marveled at his fingers, tiny toes, and all the rest.

The doctor soon came in and stood laughing, at the door
For I was up already, cleaning towels off the floor.

* * *

Many thanks to my Aunt Betty; may she be heaven blessed.
She cooked and cleaned and laundered that day so I could rest.
Many thanks to all my friends who brought casseroles and food
So I never had to cook when I wasn't in the mood.

Many thanks to Dr. O., Dr. B and Elana J.
Two doctors and a midwife who've let me have my way.
They helped build up the confidence that led to birthing Todd.
They had faith in me, we had faith in God.

One more footnote I just have to add,
A political statement that might make you mad:
When somebody has a baby too quick
They call 911 as if they are sick.
But when both are O.K., and there's danger no more
What do they go to the hospital FOR?
Everything's fine, from what I can tell.
Do you suppose it's the doctors who've something to sell?
They can't have us knowing that birth can be easy
That truly the husbands won't faint or get queasy
That birthing is not the big risk that they say
'Cause if we knew the truth, the docs would lose pay.

Happy Birthday, Todd - February 18, 1995

My Thoughts - In Ink

Inside me grows a tiny seed

Another Baby I don't need

The thought of one more mouth to feed

Stinks.

When it seems I just can't win

I think of baby's chubby chin

The sweet blue eyes, the velvet skin

So pink!

Pencil marks stretch up the wall

Measured proof that babes grow tall

The years fly past as fast as you can

Blink.

I loved to birth them I confess

And feed them often from my breast

Providing them with Natures best

Drink.

Sheila Stubbs 1995

CHAPTER 14

Afterglow

> Before I got married I had six theories about bringing up children; now I have six children and no theories.
>
> - Lord Rochester

Whether or not I really had just been "lucky" was still concerning me when I was expecting baby number six. Like many women, I had a lot of doubts and worries bothering me throughout my pregnancy. What if the baby isn't healthy? What if something goes wrong? What if my "luck" runs out?

My husband pleaded with me not to scare him again, but to promise the doctor was present for the delivery. I grudgingly agreed, insisting with equal determination that while the doctor could be present, he'd have to stay the heck away from my body and let Bert catch the baby.

The doctor said I was due next Monday, but what does he know? I predicted the baby inside was almost 10 pounds. Mother knows best.

It was Wednesday, and we were supposed to be taking my father-in-law out for supper. I was not in the mood to take an hour-long drive 40 weeks pregnant with five kids fighting in the van, only to make them sit still in a restaurant and drive home again. OK, I admit it; I was indeed *bitchy*, as my husband so nicely described it. Bert left to go for dinner with Grandpa, taking two of the kids (and in a bit of a huff, as I will nicely describe it). I should have started cooking supper for the rest of us, but decided— in a bit of a huff myself— to raise my varicose-veined legs for an hour and watch *Oprah* instead. As I climbed onto my waterbed, my water broke with an almost audible thud, wetting my maternity pants down to the knees.

It's interesting to have toddlers and teens and all in-betweens in the house when one goes into labour. At thirteen, my eldest son was somewhat embarrassed by the very fact I was pregnant: it meant his parents, as old as we were, were still "doing it." When Dr. B got my message and called me back, my son picked up the extension phone downstairs the same time I did.

"Hey, cool!" I heard him announce to all his school friends in the family room, "My mom's water just broke!"

In general, I doubt if many thirteen-year-olds know what that means. A few moments later, in about as much time as it would take Josh to explained it to them, there was a thundering of footsteps coming up the stairs as a roomful of twelve-to-fifteen-year-olds suddenly discovered something more interesting, more, like, *awesome*, than their video game. What does a woman, like, *do*, when she's, like, having a baby? They drilled me with questions.

"Are you all right? Shouldn't you lie down? Do you want me to call my dad to take you to the hospital? I could baby-sit! Are you all right? What do you want us to do? Should we call 911? Are you all right? Do you want me to call my mom?" I can understand their concern. After all, they've seen TV. They've seen the women screaming, responded to the pace of the background music, and sensed the panic of the impending emergency.

I sent them outside to play street hockey while I got to work. There was the Birth Day cake to take defrost and the champagne to chill. There were phone calls to make to let people know I was in labour, especially Bert who was on the highway somewhere, and my friend Theresa who was going to be my doula. I made a big pot of raspberry-leaf tea to drink, and started preparing the ingredients for the herbal bath. I spread an old vinyl tablecloth on the floor beside the bed to protect the carpet, and laid out some old towels, receiving blankets, and baby clothes in the bedroom. By then the contractions were already coming on pretty strong, and I needed to call my friend Theresa again, asking her to please could come over NOW! Surprised at how quickly I was progressing, she left her supper half eaten and came immediately.

It was a relief to have someone else there to talk to the kids and answer stupid questions ("Why you do dat, Mommy? What means a *contraption*, Mommy?) And I continued pacing around and around and around the kitchen table, sipping my raspberry-leaf tea in the rest between contraptions.

Bert had made the hour-long drive to his dad's place, only to be sent back home to me. I wrapped my arms around his neck, suspending my weight from him, and knew it wouldn't be long. Dr. B arrived a few minutes later. We went into the bedroom where I got ready to birth. Like young lovers hiding a secret affair, Bert waited until Dr. B wasn't looking, wrapped his arms around me and gave me a big slurpy kiss. That did the trick. I started pushing.

The only position I found comfortable was kneeling on the floor at the side of the bed – prayer position. (*Oh Dear GOD, this really HURTS*!) Dr. B wanted to examine me, but I refused, so he sat on a little stool by the bedroom door. Even though he didn't do anything, his presence irritated me. I even found his friendly chatter with my husband to be annoying and distracting; perhaps even insulting. There I was on one of the most significant moments of my life, deep in concentration, working at the most profound act in the world, bringing forth new life … and hey, how about the Blue Jays game?!

Bert put his arm around me as I sprawled my upper body over the bed. He whispered sweet things in my ear, telling me how much he loved me, and with each contraction I pushed the baby down a little more. Dr. B reminded me once again he needed to check me *before* I started pushing, because if I weren't fully dilated yet, the pushing would be ineffective. I snapped at him to stop bothering me. He sighed and shook his head. *Stubborn woman!*

Pushing was hard, and I think it was because I was inhibited by the doctor's presence. It was like trying to poop with someone watching. I wished I could have found an excuse to make him leave for even a few minutes. But after about 15 minutes of pushing - still on my knees, resting my head in my arms - I announced the baby's head would be born with the next contraction.

Dr. B popped off his stool in disbelief, and tried to check me as I knelt on the floor by the bed. I pushed his hands away as another contraction came. Dr. B wanted me <u>on</u> the bed, saying he had never delivered a baby "backwards" like that. Too bad; I couldn't move, it hurt too much. Dr. B put his hand on the baby's head to support it as it emerged, and it hurt.

"LEAVE IT ALONE!" I yelled at him, "DON'T TOUCH IT!" He tried to show Bert what to do; how to support the baby's head. "GET AWAY! LEAVE IT!" I hollered, and pushed away the doctor's hands.

"But I'm not doing anything!" he protested, "I'm just—"

"Well STOP IT!" I yelled at him, shoving him away. (Apparently I get a little cranky in labour!) Theresa and my eight-year-old daughter were in the kitchen giggling, listening to this entire drama.

Dr. B left me alone - mainly because I was slapping him - but he got down on his hands and knees behind me, bending over to see what I wouldn't let him touch. Bert bent over for a peek too, the two of them on their hands and knees, heads cocked like a couple of mechanics checking under the car for a leak.

"PUSH!" they both yelled, looking at an upside-down scrunched-up little purple face. Like I wasn't already?

Bert guided the baby out as he slid to the floor. Dr. B immediately jumped in between us to tie the cord, and it was at that moment I really noticed the intrusion. Bert noticed it too, and we glanced at each other, and understood.

How wonderful and sweet those moments had been when our previous baby was born. Even though Bert had been somewhat shaken by having to play midwife unexpectedly, we had been alone for almost half an hour before the doctor arrived. Our deepest emotions had gushed out uninhibited, laughing and crying in joy. It was so intimate - simply my husband and me and the baby we made together and birthed together. Just us, and then our children joined us to marvel at their new sibling who had just come from my body as they had. Our new baby was welcomed into the family on a cold February morning surrounded only by those who loved him. No outsiders had intruded on the sacredness of the moment, and it belonged to our family alone.

This time however, Dr. B had the cord tied and cut faster than you can say "procedure." He had not only taken that moment to separate the baby from me, but also me from Bert; his body physically between us. The doctor's presence had subtly affected our relationships at that moment. We had done it a better way, and now we knew the difference.

I sent my daughter to fetch her brothers, who took one quick look at the new baby and said, "Cool! But… can we go finish our hockey game now?" I had a quick shower then joined everyone in the kitchen for the celebration.

Since I had been labouring over the supper hour, a neighbour who owed us a favour brought two extra-large pizzas. They were amazed to see a woman sitting in the kitchen eating pizza and cake and drinking champagne within an hour after giving birth! I was smugly proud to think I managed to avoid having even one single vaginal exam through an entire pregnancy, labour, and delivery. We discovered a crowd of neighbourhood kids had gathered on our front yard. The trees had been decorated with baby-blue balloons! The road in front of our house was brightly coloured in chalk messages! I wouldn't allow any of the crowd into the house to sneeze on my newborn, but when I took the baby to the front window they cheered!

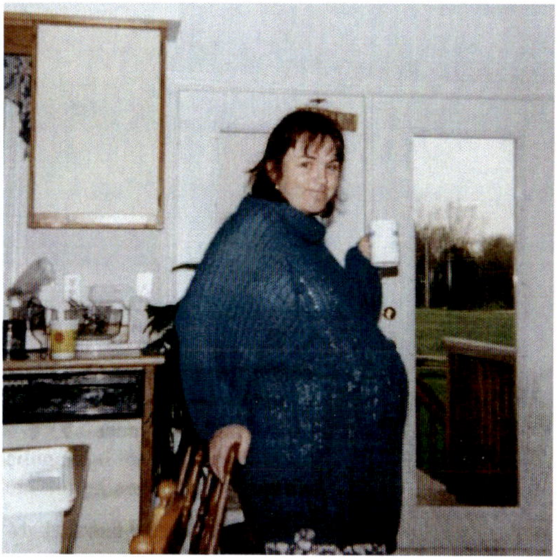

5pm – In labour, sipping red-raspberry-leaf-tea between contractions.

The Birth Day Cake is thawing for the party.

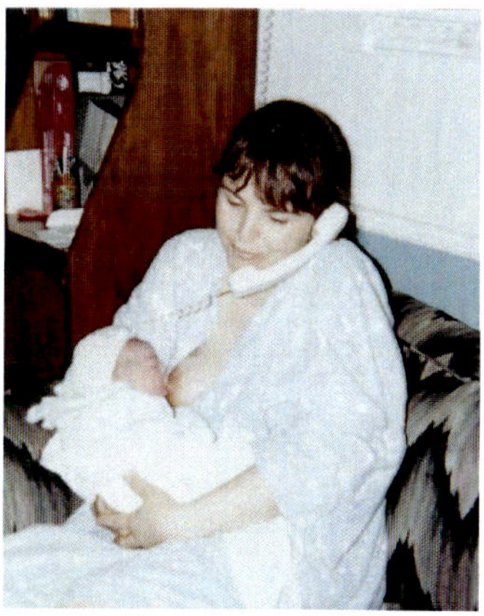

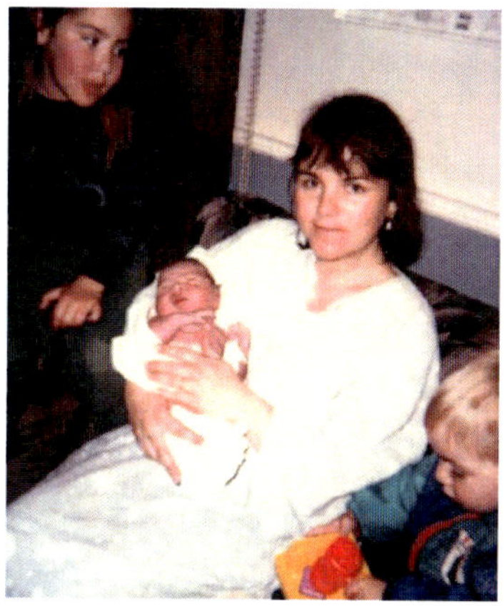

8pm- Celebrating in the kitchen with pizza and champagne and Birth Day Cake and phone calls to share the news! Baby's siblings are playing with their new Birth Day Party toys.

The scales we had borrowed weren't very precise, but indicated the baby was about 10 pounds (just as I had predicted!) which is accurate enough for documents. However, he was only 18 inches long, which also could explain why it felt like giving birth to a bag of potatoes.

Afterglow

If we ever have another baby, we will guard our privacy with a vengeance. Bert says we aren't going to have any more. Come to think of it, he said that just before the last two were born. It's just that the previous birth – the one we had done by ourselves -- was so... so *romantic*. There had been such a beautiful, smooth flow to the labour. There was no disruption, no interference, no outsider involvement, no need for someone to check my progress, and nobody had to tell me when and how to push. The beauty was in the absence of all these distractions. We'd had the freedom to enjoy the awesome power of giving birth uninhibited as both an emotional and spiritual climax in all its fullness. Blissful over our accomplishment, in awe of the beauty and incredible power of birth, we had basked in the afterglow of our own miracle.

Along with endless teasing about his midwifery skills, Bert was regarded as quite a hero by friends and coworkers who were amazed he could deliver his own baby with nothing but a single white shoelace for tying the cord. He smugly accepted his status. But he knows, and I know — the way we shared the birth of our fifth baby was really beautifully simple... and simply beautiful.

This book would never have been written without the services of the following folks who provided uninterrupted blocks of time for writing.

Walt Disney

Barney

Elliot Moose

The late Fred Rogers

Sharon, Lois, & Bramm

Inspector Gadget

Arthur Reid

Tinky Winky, Dipsy, Lala, Po

Notes

[1] "Strathroy Police... We Deliver!" The Age Dispatch, Strathroy, Ont., November 1, 1995, p. 11.

[2] "NATURAL CHILDBIRTH.... this mother of nine delivers her own babies" Look Magazine, November 13, 1956

[3] Ontario Ministry of Health, Report on the Task Force on the Implementation of Midwifery in Ontario, p. 220; 1987.

[4] Cynthia Carver MD, Patient Beware, (Prentice-Hall 1984), p. 169.

[5] Patricia Cloyd Carter; Come Gently, Sweet Lucina, Titusville, Florida, 1957, p. 229.

[6] ibid., page 227-28.

[7] Carolyn Flint, in an address at the International Conference on waterbirth, London England, as quoted in Compleat Mother , Vol. 40., Winter 1995.

[8] The Compleat Mother, Spring '98.

[9] Carter, Come Gently Sweet Lucina, Titusville, Florida, 1957, pg. 58

[10] Sheila Kitzinger, speaking at the Third International Homebirth Conference in Stockholm, Sweden, October 3, 1997, as quoted in Compleat Mother, Spring 1998.

[11] Cynthia Carver MD, Patient Beware, (Prentice-Hall 1984), p. 153

[12] ibid., page 152-153

[13] Adelle Davis, Let's Have Healthy Children, (Signet, 1972), p. 124-6

[14] The Perinatal Education Program of Eastern Ontario for Health and Welfare Canada, Present Patterns & Trends in Infant Feeding In Canada, 1990. p. 7.

[15] Jelliffe & Jelliffe, Human Milk in the Modern World, (Oxford University Press, 1978.)

[16] Dr. Jack Newman, MD, FRCPC, Still More Breastfeeding Myths, Handout # 13, Myth #15, March 1993

---

[17] Marshall Klaus and Kennell, John, Maternal-Infant Bonding: *The Impact of Early Separation or Loss on Family Development*, (C.V. Mosby Co. 1976)

[18] Dr. Cynthia Carver, MD. Patient Beware (Prentice-Hall Canada 1994),p.41

[19] Babette Francis, B.Sc., Successful Lactation and Women's Sexuality, Reprint no. 148. (La Leche League International, August 1978)reprinted from *The Journal of Tropical Pediatrics and Environmental Child Health,* Vol. 22, No. 4 August 1976. Based on a paper presented at National Conference on Women's Health in a Changing Society: Univ. of Queensland, St. Lucia, Brisbane, August 27, 1975.

[20] Perinatal Education Program of Eastern Ontario, p.4

[21] The Womanly Art of Breastfeeding; La Leche League International, 35th Anniversary Edition 1991, p. 117.

[22] ibid. pg. 358

[23] Michel Odent, MD; *Sexuality is More Than Sex*; Compleat Mother Magazine, Winter 1993

[24] Lynn M. Griesemer, Unassisted Homebirth - An Act of Love, (Terra Publishing, Charleston, SC 1998)p.46

[25] Robert S. Mendelsohn, MD, Confessions of a Medical Heretic, 1979, p. 150

[26] Marian Tompson, "Custom-Made Delivery" in Safe Alternatives in Childbirth, (NAPSAC, 1976), p.141,143

[27] Ontario Ministry of Health, Report of the Task Force on the Implementation of Midwifery in Ontario, 1987, p 33.

[28] Grantly Dick-Read, Childbirth Without Fear (Harper & Row, 1944, 1953, Renewed 1972 by Jessica Dick-Read).

[29] "*Prenatal ultrasound can be wrong: study,*" Oxford Review, Woodstock, Ont., Saturday, November 01, 1998, p. 19.

[30] Ontario Ministry of Health, p.109.

[31] Lewis E, Mehl, MD, "Statistical Outcomes of Homebirths in the US: Current Status," in Safe Alternatives in Childbirth, ed. by David & Lee Stewart, (N.A.P.S.A.C. [National Association of Parents and Professionals for Safe Alternatives in Childbirth] 1976) p.73-99.

[32] Jessica Mitford, The American Way of Birth, (Dutton,1992), p.31

[33] Henci Goer, The Thinking Woman's Guide to a Better Birth, (Perigree, 1999) p.202

[34] Dr. Robert S. Mendelsohn, MD, How to Raise a Healthy Child in Spite of Your Doctor, (Ballantyne, 1984) p. 48.

[35] William's Obstetrics, 15th Edition, 1976, Prentice-Hall

[36] William's Obstetrics, 20th Edition, 1997, Appleton & Lange Stamford, Connecticut

[37] Ontario Ministry of Health, Report of the Task Force on the Implementation of Midwifery in Ontario, 1987, p. 198.

[38] ibid., p. 35 footnote.

[39] ibid., p. 30.

[40] ibid., p. 209.

[41] ibid., p. 098-199.

[42]Percy E. Ryberg, MD, Health, Sex, and Birth Control, (Anchor Press, 1940).

[43] Dr, Willial H. Hazlett, "The Male Factor in Obstetrics", *Child and Family*, Fall 1974

[44] Ontario Ministry of Health, Report of the Task Force on the Implementation of Midwifery in Ontario, 1987, p,218

[45] ibid.

[46] Ontario Ministry of Health, Footnote #119, p. 231.

[61] Michele Harrison, A Woman in Residence, (New York: Random House, 1982)

[48] Mendelsohn, Confessions p.221-2

[63] Robert S. Mendelsohn, MD, Mal(e) Practice: How Doctors Manipulate Women, (Contemporary 1981), p. 139-40.

[64] Mendelsohn, Mal(e) Practice, p. 139-40.

[51] Mendelsohn, Confessions... p. 152-3.

[52] Wagner, Marsden, Born in the USA, page78.

[53] Nancy W, Cohen and Lois J. Estner, Silent Knife, (Bergin & Garvey 1983), p. 180.

[54] Mendelsohn, Confessions... p. 155.

[39] Mendelsohn, Mal(e)Practice page 168-70.

[56] ibid., page 152.

Notes

[57] Henci Goer, The Thinking Woman's Guide to a Better Birth, (Perigree 1999), p. 158.

[58] Williams Obstetrics 20th Edition, © 1997 by Appleton & Lange Stamford, Connecticut, p. 343

[59] Mendelsohn, How to Raise a Healthy Child…, p.255

[60] Michele Harrison, A Woman in Residence (New York, Random House, 1982)

[61] ibid., page 147.

[62] Laura Kaplan Shanley, Unassisted Childbirth, (Bergin & Garvey 1994), p. 140

[63] "*Infant Care*: We've been all wrong for years about umbilical cords," The London Free Press, Saturday November 2, 1994; p. D10.

[64] Mendelsohn, MalePractice p. 143-144.

[65] Mary Jane Egan, "Say So long to Hospital Nurseries", The London Free Press, London, Ontario; Saturday March 4, 2000, page A3.

[66] See the "Breast Crawl" video at www.breastcrawl.org.

[67] Mendelsohn, How to Raise a Healthy Child… in Spite of Your Doctor, (Ballantyne, 1984), page 19.

[68] Catherine Young, Compleat Mother Magazine, Spring 1998, Volume 49, Editorial.

[69] William H, Hazlett, MD, "The Male Factor Hn Obstetrics" Child & Family, Fall 1967,

[70] Dr. Carolyn Rawlings, speaking at La Leche League's 1983 Conference, available on tape from LLLI.

[71] Thames Valley Midwives(London, Ontario) website: http://tvm.on.ca

[72] Dr. James Dobson, Focus on The Family Radio broadcast. Available on tape from Focus on the Family, P.O. Box 9800, Station Terminal, Vancouver BC, V6B 4G3.

[73] Marilyn Moran, *Birth as an Act of Love*, Mothering Magazine, Summer 1981.

[74] Marilyn A Moran; Birth and The Dialogue of Love, (New Nativity Press 1981), p. 226.

[75] Deborah Tanzer, Why Natural Childbirth?, (1972, Schocken),p.168

[76]Marilyn A. Moran, Attachment or Loss Within Marriage: The Effect of the Medical Model of Birthing on the Marital Bond of Love; Pre- and Perinatal Psychology Journal, 6(4), Summer 1992:265.

[77] Marilyn A. Moran, Pleasurable Husband/Wife Childbirth ...The real consummation of married love; (New Nativity Press 1997), page 52.

[78] Come Gently Sweet Lucina, 1957, Titusville, Florida, p. 56, 57.

[79] Carter, p. 201.

[80] Moran, M.A., Attachment or loss within marriage: The effect of the medical model of birthing on the marital bond of love. . (1992) Pre- & Perinatal Psychology Journal, 6(4), 265-280.

[81] Ashley Montague, Touching: The Human Significance of the Skin, (Harper & Row 1978), p.255.

[82] Jean Leidloff, The Continuum Concept, Addison Wessley1977, p.158.

[83] Laura Kaplan Shanley, Unassisted Childbirth, 1994, Bergin & Garvey (introduction)

[84] Robbie Davis-Floyd, Birth as an American Rite of Passage, 1992, Univ. of California Press, Berkely, p. 69-70.

[85] I read this in an interesting old book I borrowed from the Amway lady. The book described how to pick a good wife (including checking her teeth and her hips,) how to deflower her, and other related items for the 19th century man. I lost the name of the Amway lady and therefore, the reference. Go find her in Strathroy, ON.

[86] Laura Kaplan Shanley, Unassisted Childbirth, 1994, Bergin & Garvey, p.112.

[87] Shanley, p.9.

[88] Moran, Pleasurable Husband/Wife Childbirth, p.85-6.

[89] Ina May Gaskin, Spiritual Midwifery, 1978, The Book Publishing Company, The Farm, Tennessee, p. 349.

[90] ibid., p. 444.

[91] Carter, p. 329-331,

[92] Lynn M. Griesemer, Unassisted Homebirth - An act of Love (Terra Publishing 1988), page 260.

[93] Griesemer, p. 46.

[94] Lester D. Hazell, Commonsense Childbirth, Berkley Publishing Corporation, p. 102, 209.

Notes

[95] Laura O'Banion "Delivering Labor in the 20th Century." 1987 Paper in lieu of Master's Thesis, Dept. of Anthropology, Univ. of Illinois at Urbana Champaign.

[96] Ok I admit it: Alena James is one of my pennames. We can't have people knowing that this nice Sunday School teacher would write such a story, can we?